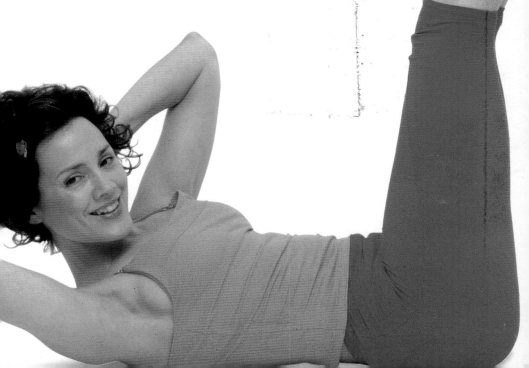

PERSONAL TRAINER
PILATES & YOGA

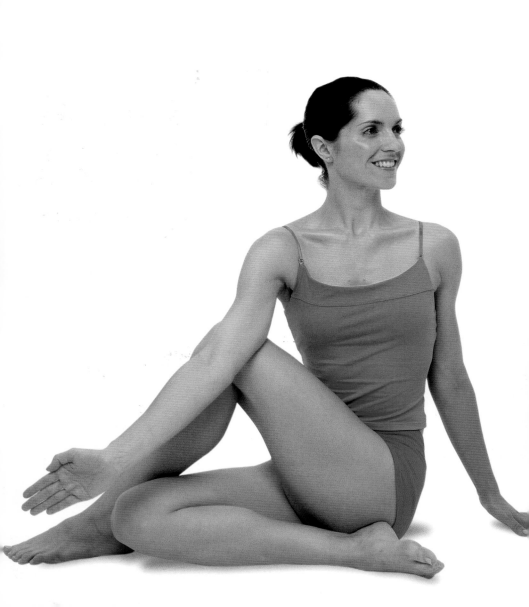

PERSONAL TRAINER
PILATES & YOGA

JILL EVERETT

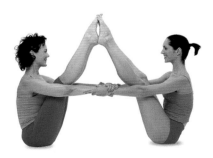

CARLTON
BOOKS

With love, respect and gratitude to my teachers and to my students.

THIS IS A CARLTON BOOK

Text copyright © 2003 Breathe Enterprises Ltd
Design and special photography copyright © 2003
Carlton Books Limited

First published in 2003
This edition published in 2010 by
by Carlton Books Limited
20 Mortimer Street
London W1T 3JW

A CIP catalogue record for this book is available from the British Library.
ISBN 978 1 84732 475 7

Printed and bound in Dubai

It is important to consult your doctor before commencing any
exercise programme. This is particularly the case if you have a
medical condition (including, but not limited to, abnormal blood
pressure or a back injury), have had surgery recently or are
pregnant and, even then, you should only undertake these
programmes with a well-trained teacher. All instructions and
warnings given in this book should be read carefully. This book
is not intended to replace personal instruction or professional
medical advice. The contraindications/warnings listed for some
poses are guidelines only.

The author and publisher have made every effort to ensure that
all information is correct and up to date at the time of publication.
Neither the author nor the publisher can accept responsibility for,
or shall be liable for, any accident, injury, loss or damage
(including any consequential loss) that results from using the
ideas, information, procedures or advice offered in this book.

Editorial Manager: Judith More
Art Director: Penny Stock
Project Editor: Lisa Dyer
Copy Editors: Jane Donovan
and Sarah Sears
Design: DW Design
Special Photography:
Anna Stevenson
Make-up Artist: Neusa Neves
Production Controller:
Lisa French

contents

foreword by Dr Jennifer Golay Bengston

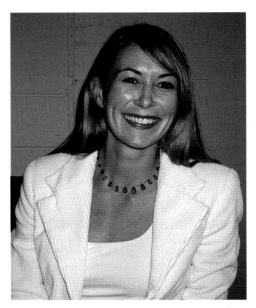

As a chiropractor in a busy multidisciplinary health-care practice, I regularly treat patients who are unable to fully enjoy their lives because of chronic inhibiting musculo-skeletal (muscle, bone and joint) complaints. Many of these patients complain of back, leg, neck and arm pain or headaches, resulting from a recent injury causing a chronic pain problem or aggravating an old injury. Typically, after an initial course of chiropractic treatment, the patients that fulfil the recommended stretches and exercises recover significantly sooner than those who refrain. The patient who becomes 'actively' involved in their own rehabilitation tends to report less subjective pain levels, has increased range of motion, and increased stability and strength, and – most importantly – returns to activities they enjoy and improved health.

I believe that having a healthy spine begins with performing exercises that increase strength and flexibility. Two very effective forms of exercise to achieve this are pilates and yoga. This combined programme provides an exemplary avenue for strengthening the spine and battling instability and weakness, which can be the culprit in many musculo-skeletal complaints. Working deep postural muscles develops core strength, which is integral to body stability, strength and balance. These muscles will support you in everyday activities, such as standing, walking and sitting, preventing the slumping or slouching that usually occur with exhaustion or because of poor posture.

We live in an age where most of our time is spent in a 'sitting' posture, whether we are working at a desk, eating a meal or travelling to and from work. We tend to hold our bodies in chronic postures that compromise our optimal health. These daily activities contribute to a weakening of our bodies – perhaps producing a posture where the shoulders roll forward and the front of the body sinks back, shortens and caves in, with a rounded spine. To reverse this process, we need to support the spine.

In the following pages, focus on the subtlety of each movement and understand the pose required before you rush off to make the movement. Visualize – picture what you are about to do in your head – and then hold the starting position to feel the movement before you do it. Having the correct posture as you exercise will carry over into your everyday life. All the muscles of the body have a memory and it will soon become easier for you to stand or sit up straight without feeling pain and exhaustion at the end of the day. Those among my patients who practise yoga or pilates routinely seem to maintain the improvements they have gained. They say that, after following the exercise plan for a while, it feels abnormal to slouch or sit with round shoulders .

This book's regime presents a great programme for the prevention of pain and the creation of a healthy and strong body. In addition, it will reduce and alleviate chronic pain, and leave you revived and feeling good all over! Before undertaking any new exercise plan, please consult your healthcare professional or chiropractor. This book is designed for people without serious injury; it isn't advisable for pregnant women to use it without supervision.

introduction by Jill Everett

If this book has managed to present itself to you, then you may be ready to take your relationship with health, your mind, body and soul, a bit further. Are you ready to feel better, mentally and physically? Then this book is for you. It's for anyone who is searching for a connection of mind, body and soul, for inner peace, for inner and outer strength, for freedom from pain. It's for anyone who wants to re-claim their body, to experience the sheer joy of movement, to feel the lightness that only comes from a strong, healthy, supple body. Wouldn't it be great to feel that any physical task could be done simply and effortlessly? Or even to look forward to physical activity rather than dread it? Just to have a few hours free of pain may be enough for one person, while another wants physical perfection, and another self-realization! We are here for different reasons but we can all benefit from simple common-sense truths that open our bodies and our hearts. Health is freedom – when we restore balance to the body we open ourselves to the wonders of life.

In the next chapter, you'll learn the history, philosophy, and heart and soul of this fusion programme. You'll also learn about the body to better understand how medically sound the combined approach is. Then we'll go through some essential principles. This is a precision method focusing on correct alignment, breath, flowing movement and control from the deep core abdominals – with a focused mind, in a relaxed manner. Without these principles you are merely doing a body-conditioning routine and you will not achieve the same results. Stay focused for your first few months and the correct habits will become second nature and you will begin to feel more relaxed during the classes. Continuity and perseverance are required. This training will bring a freedom to the body, necessary for it to function properly. Once you are really stable in your body you can further challenge it with movements requiring flexibility and strength and it will respond without strain and injury. And you know you are advanced when you can do all of this calmly, breathing easily – with a smile!

Listen to your body. The golden rule is 'strength before flexibility'. I am aware of many students' desire to do very advanced exercises and postures before they are ready. These are empty gymnastic movements without understanding, and do not respect the body. Be patient. Both pilates and yoga look in great detail at the progress of the individual practice and correct alignment of the body to strengthen muscles, stabilize joints and improve, not injure, the body! Carefully read each chapter before you begin the exercises. My method works and the practice transforms – that's why it's so popular! So get busy, put your heart into it and enjoy the liberation it brings. It could change your life!

the spirit of yoga & pilates

As beginning students of yoga and pilates we're often looking for better posture, increased flexibility, smaller hips, or toned stomachs. Or maybe we're interested because our health has deteriorated or because we feel our lives are out of control and we can't stand the stress anymore. We're usually looking for even more than that, but we may not know exactly what it is we are searching for. When people ask me why I choose to practise pilates or yoga, I say because it's fun! Because it is fun to twist and stretch and move! Practising yoga and pilates also allows me to be me, to better realize who I really am, and it shows me how I can bring peace to my relationships with the world.

By building a strong body, and learning how to relax and calm the nervous system, we free the mind and allow ourselves time for self-reflection. To many people, who have busy lives juggling work and children, this may seem an unattainable luxury, but it's actually a real necessity. If we don't have a strong body and a focused mind, how can we begin to contemplate carrying out our intentions and maintaining our values in a world which sometimes seems increasingly at odds with the life we really want to live? So in yoga the ultimate goal is the direct realization of who we really are, and in pilates we aim for balance and control – balance of body and mind, balance in our lives, balance in our breathing, and control of the mind and body. We could go on for pages and pages just to begin to define yoga and pilates more fully, but it's much better for you to learn by first-hand experience!

An overview of yoga practices

It seems sensible to start with what we know of yoga in modern life: the deep stretching, the breathing techniques, the meditation. In fact, this is just a tiny fragment of what yoga really is; it's not the full picture. Yoga is a whole way of life, developed thousands of years ago, an education for the body, mind and spirit. It's said to be the art of right living. Only in recent times has yoga been more associated with the physical postures; in ancient times it was the meditative practices that were thought to have much more prominence.

Over the centuries yoga has developed in four very different strands. Karma yoga is the path of selfless service, followed by those such as Mother Teresa of Calcutta. Jnana yoga, in contrast, is much more an intellectual approach to spiritual evolution and is often practised by philosophers and sociologists, for example. Bhakti yoga is the devotional path expressed by singers, musicians, chanters and others who express their art in a devotional way. Raja yoga, meanwhile, is based on a more practical system of concentration and mind control, manifested in the meditation and the asanas, that we practise in a yoga class. It's raja yoga that we will focus on in this book, because raja yoga teaches that a healthy body, steady posture, breath regulation, right living and the withdrawal of the senses lead to the ultimate goal of self-realization.

The father of yoga in modern times is the great Tirumalai Krishnamacharya, who revolutionized yoga for the twentieth century. Born in Mysore in southern India in 1888, into a family who could trace its lineage back to a famous ninth-century sage, Krishnamacharya studied the vedic yoga texts from the age of 12, and he later went on to university to study Sanskrit, logic and grammar. Having spent many more years with his teachers, Krishnamacharya opened a yoga school in Mysore in 1924. His yoga teaching was unique because he attended to the individual, adjusting all practices to meet his students' personal needs, rather than making the individual adjust to meet the requirements of yoga. The way he approached spreading his message was unique too. He toured around India with a troupe of boys performing amazing gymnastic-style yogic feats, because he knew that if he got people's attention, he would then be able to enrol them as students, thereby drawing them back to the real message of yoga. Krishnamacharya never saw yoga simply as a physical practice, but much more about reaching God. He was also the first teacher to teach a woman, and a foreign woman at that –

Indra Devi, who went on to become one of the most famous teachers in the West, with many top Hollywood movie stars, including Greta Garbo, among her students.

Krishnamacharya knew that yoga had to adapt to the modern world – or it would vanish. Krishnamacharya's students have become the most influential yoga teachers in the world today: BKS Iyengar, K Pattabhi Jois, Indra Devi and his own son TKV Desikachar. These four teachers all have very different practices: Pattabhi Jois is the father of modern ashtanga yoga; BKS Iyengar is the father of iyengar yoga; Indra Devi teaches a gentle form of Krishnamacharya's ashtanga yoga; and TKV Desikachar is the father of vini yoga.

The Joseph Pilates method

Pilates is a physical exercise technique that incorporates mind and body and also nurtures the spirit. It was created by Joseph Pilates, who was born in Germany in 1880. Pilates suffered many physical ailments as a child, such as rickets and asthma, so he tirelessly experimented with his own frail physique in his quest to attain a strong healthy body. He practised gymnastics, skiing, diving, martial arts, circus acrobatics, yoga, boxing and many other body-conditioning methods. By the age of 14 Pilates had so improved his body that he was posing as a model for anatomical drawings. Pilates was a young adult at the beginning of the twentieth century when physical-fitness crazes had become very popular and new knowledge of the human mind and body had been discovered. It was an exciting time. Cars and telephones had been invented, modern living was fast paced and stress had begun to take its toll on the average big-city dweller. By the 1920s, when Harvard set up its Harvard Fatigue Laboratory to research the effects of exercise on the body, Pilates was already talking about ways of combating unnatural physical fatigue and nervous strain caused by modern life.

In 1923 he moved to New York City and set up his studio, where he trained clients from all walks of life: dancers, writers, actors and industrialists. He was often involved in debates of the day on poor diet, badly designed furniture and inadequate, unbalanced exercise fads, which, he observed, contributed to the flat feet and overly curved spines he saw around him. The pilates method was rich in balance. Pilates had been inspired by Eastern and Western philosophies to create something new and exciting. Of the utmost importance in the pilates method was the link between physical and mental wellbeing. Pilates was also very influenced by yoga, as is illustrated in his use of specific breathing techniques, mental focus, extreme flexibility demonstrations and flow. His love of gymnastics enhanced the physicality of the pilates method and he developed a system which promoted flexibility, strength, stamina and a relaxed sense of focus and wellbeing. By balancing the actions of the joints and muscles Pilates had developed a near-perfect fitness system which still stands today, a century later, as a successful blueprint for structural fitness.

Joseph Pilates created many different movements in his method, some of which could be performed on the floor, with no equipment. These were known as mat work. Other exercises involved working on pieces of equipment, using springs and pulleys, and these could then be combined with the floor exercises. The mat work, comprising 34 exercises, is the original movement system and is commonly referred to as the 'full mat', or 'classical pilates'. Pilates developed his method at a time when many people were involved in physical labour, workers were often used to standing and people walked. In today's society, where not many people are likely to walk for more than 10 minutes a day, or stand upright for more than 10 to 20 minutes at a time, a beginner will find these exercises quite challenging.

Pilates teaching techniques

Most people today generally don't have the core strength to begin a classical pilates programme with the original 34 mat exercises, so other methods have been developed in recent years which break down the original exercises into easier sequences with the same goals as the originals. This has been a successful way to bring the benefits of the pilates method to people who, through lack of correct exercise, injury, poor health or any number of other reasons, have physical limitations.

I use many pilates prep exercises here and some classical pilates

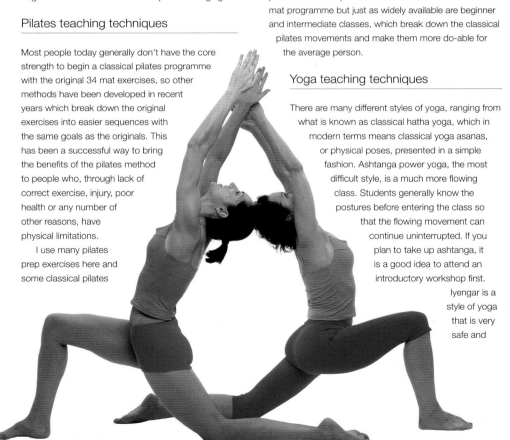

exercises as well. I combine these with yoga postures to create an amazing flowing sequence that should challenge, inspire, relax and strengthen you. Pilates and yoga classes are now offered separately all over the world. You may see names attached to the various methods and wonder about the differences between them. Generally speaking, pilates classes are either group classes, led by one teacher, or machine-based studio classes using equipment – in a pilates-style gym. It will be possible to find a pilates class that offers the classical full-mat programme but just as widely available are beginner and intermediate classes, which break down the classical pilates movements and make them more do-able for the average person.

Yoga teaching techniques

There are many different styles of yoga, ranging from what is known as classical hatha yoga, which in modern terms means classical yoga asanas, or physical poses, presented in a simple fashion. Ashtanga power yoga, the most difficult style, is a much more flowing class. Students generally know the postures before entering the class so that the flowing movement can continue uninterrupted. If you plan to take up ashtanga, it is a good idea to attend an introductory workshop first.

Iyengar is a style of yoga that is very safe and

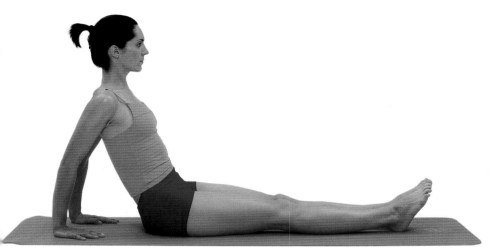

thorough, making it good for building strength and for learning the postures. Though he practised most of the same classical postures employed by all other yoga methods, it was BKS Iyengar who pioneered the use of props, such as foam blocks and bricks, belts, ropes, bolsters, wooden tables, chairs and other toys to help people into postures they could not otherwise manage safely. This made yoga accessible to far more people, and also made it therapeutic for injuries, illnesses and other physical limitations. BKS Iyengar still teaches at his centre in Pune, India, with his daughter Geeta and son Prashant.

Indra Devi's gentle flowing practice is classical ashtanga with an additional devotional element and involves a small meditation in each posture. It is also very focused on the breath with each posture. TKV Desikachar, son of Krishnamacharya, pioneered the vini yoga method taught by many of his European students. Desikachar's vini yoga stresses the need to adapt the teaching of yoga to the individual and also places great emphasis on linking the breath with the various asanas – excellent practice for all levels. Desikachar still teaches at the Krisnamacharya Centre in Mysore, India.

Scaravelli yoga is another excellent method that is suitable for beginners. Vanda Scaravelli, its pioneer, taught yoga well into her 80s and stressed the gentle approach to achieve and maintain overall health and a naturally supple spine at any age. A student of BKS Iyengar for many years, Scaravelli has recently died and Scaravelli yoga is now taught mainly in Europe by her

students. Sivananda yoga is a yogic practice based on simple living and high thinking, incorporating proper exercise, proper breathing, proper relaxation and a proper vegetarian diet. Positive thinking and meditation complete this full programme for a better life. Students of sivananda yoga may take classes in yoga ashrams the world over and can also attend classes on a residential basis, staying in the ashrams for various lengths of time.

The combined approach

I believe that in my programme I have combined the best of all worlds! I have put together a regime that represents a full body, mind and soul workout for a beginner, progressing to an intermediate level.

Through years of experience as a teacher and as a student of some of the world's most amazing teachers, I have learned what I struggle with and also what many others struggle with. My students have been some of my best teachers as it is through them that I have tried and tested my methods. My own physical fitness comes from hard work and many long hours of intensive training, so I do understand about pain and limitations!

I have been lucky to have had the benefit of some spectacular teachers. I am hugely grateful to all of them for inspiring me, teaching me everything they knew, rehabilitating and caring for me, and making things fun! I hope that some of their magic has rubbed off on me and that I can do the same for you through my book.

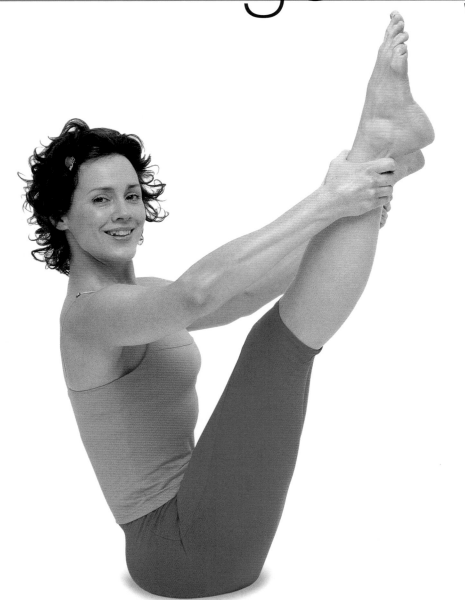

started

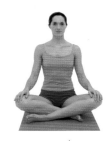

Before you begin any exercises, make sure you have read through this entire section and learned the principles described. The fusion of pilates and yoga is a precise form of movement, and you may find instructions in this section that you are not familiar with, even if you have practised yoga before. Learn the terminology, practise engaging the pelvic floor, find your correct postural alignment, learn about your spine and try the meditation and breathing exercises. Once you can demonstrate neutral pelvis/neutral spine, find your pelvic floor engagement and practise lateral breathing, then you are ready to move onto the exercise programmes.

how to use this book

Please start from the beginning and read all the chapters before you begin. My fusion of pilates and yoga is a very precise method and is different from most other forms of exercise you may already have practised. It is especially important that you understand the 'getting started' information before you begin the exercise programmes. It is good to start with some brief breathing and meditation exercises to enable you to connect with yourself easily and ready yourself for the programme that follows (see pages 20–3).

The pre-exercise movement programme lists six exercises aimed at those who are new to exercise, or who just feel that they would like to start slowly. Once you can easily complete this sequence without feeling fatigued or unsteady, you can then progress to the warm-up sequence combined with the beginner's programme. When you are able to complete the beginner's programme easily with no strain or fatigue, you can then progress to the warm-up sequence followed by the intermediate programme. I have included three mini sets for a brief but balanced workout, targeted to boost energy, to destress and to strengthen the back. These can be performed any time, in combination with one of the other sequences in the book or on their own.

It's a good idea to see if you can find a pilates or yoga class in your area to get some supervision from a qualified teacher. This will help your understanding of what you are doing and will speed up your progress. If you are unsure of where to find a class, just search the internet under 'pilates' or 'yoga' in the name of your town. Alternatively, purchase a yoga magazine; these usually include listings of yoga centres and contact numbers for organizations and classes.

Injuries and pregnancy

This programme has been written for a person in normal physical condition with no injuries. If you have an old or ongoing injury, please check with your doctor before you do any of the exercises. Every injury is different so it is impossible to say generally what can be beneficial or detrimental to you. If you feel pain, stop what you are doing. Every exercise should be performed pain-free. Effort and hard work are one thing and strain, which can cause damage, is another.

This programme is not designed for pregnant women. Pilates can be great for pregnancy, but only if you have been practising it regularly before your pregnancy, and if you are supervised by a teacher who knows how to teach pilates for pregnancy. Pregnancy is not an ideal time to start any new form of exercise and pilates in particular works the abdominals so strongly that even a normal programme would not be a good idea for a pregnant beginner. But pilates is definitely great as part of your post-natal regime. You can begin as soon as you get clearance from your doctor at your post-natal checkup.

General advice

Do not eat for two hours before exercising and wear something you can bend and stretch comfortably in. Dancewear or clothes that are close-fitting are best, as they make it easier for you to see what your body is doing if you look in a mirror to check something. Exercise using a thick, non-slip yoga mat. This will protect the spine and also acts as a good stable base for standing exercises as your feet won't slip. It is best to work in bare feet. Practise this programme at least three or four times a week. It is best to practise every day, especially at the beginning, to familiarize yourself with the method and retain what you learn from each class.

guidelines

Both pilates and yoga have some basic ground rules with which you must familiarize yourself, as I refer to them throughout the exercise sequences. Once you can find alignment and neutral pelvis/neutral spine for all positions – standing, sitting, kneeling, lying on your back, side or tummy – you should master the pelvic-floor engagement and breathing. Please put some time into getting these basics right; when you understand them you're ready to move on to the exercise programmes.

The eight principles of Pilates

These principles should be employed in each exercise:
1 **Concentration** Be present. Forget the job, or whatever. Pay attention, be aware and focus on what you are doing.
2 **Centring** Every movement you make comes from your centre. Try reaching for a cup and feel your abdominals engage to balance you. A strong stable centre is the basis of everything in pilates. Engage your centre before you move.
3 **Flow** Fluid, elegant motion replaces the jerky bounces of other exercise techniques. Observe and smooth out moves. As you become more advanced one exercise also flows into the next.
4 **Breath** The breath connects the mind and body: breathing is necessary! You're breathing all the time so learn how to breathe better. Don't hold your breath when you find something difficult. Keep the breathing pattern going and see how it helps a movement – deep, full breaths, inhaling through the nose, exhaling through the mouth.
5 **Control** Pilates called his method 'contrology'. The mind controls every muscle during the workout. No random movements please!
6 **Alignment** Check your alignment before you start each exercise. You will learn to 'find neutral pelvis/neutral spine', when the skeleton is in the correct position from head to toe with no tension in any of the joints, so that as you build muscle, you won't develop any that will hold you in an incorrect posture. You will need to learn what is correct alignment for sitting, kneeling on all fours, standing, lying on your back, side and front.
7 **Relaxation** Our exercises are performed in a relaxed manner. If you have no strength to begin with, this may sound difficult, but you will build strength gradually and then see how you can perform the movements with ease.
8 **Stamina** You will build up stamina slowly. Don't try anything too difficult too soon, but do challenge yourself. Develop body awareness, know your 'safe range', then trust your judgement. A pilates workout is challenging, especially the complex sequences; you will need stamina!

Alignment and neutral pelvis /neutral spine

To begin exercising you need to know how to find your neutral pelvis/neutral spine in a standing position, lying down on your back, lying face-down, lying on your side and kneeling on all fours.

standing alignment
1 Stand with your feet parallel, hip-width apart, with your weight evenly on both feet. Gently lift through your inner arches, inner ankles, knees and the front of your thighs. Lift your hip bones, and balance the pelvis by taking the navel back to the spine, pulling the tailbone down towards the floor. The spine is long; pull up through the top of your head – as if balloons are lifting you up to the sky.
2 The chest lifts, the shoulder blades move down towards your waist. Your arms are at your sides, facing forwards at elbows, wrists and palms. The neck is long and the chin parallel to the floor; look to the front. The legs are long and open, the knees softly bent – don't force them backwards.
3 From a side-view we see that the head is directly above the shoulders, ribcage, hips, knees and feet. A plumbline could cut through the centre of the ear, neck, upper arm, ribcage, just in front of the hip bone, just behind the knee cap and just in front of the ankle bone. Use this upright alignment in your everyday life!

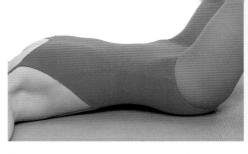

This close-up of the torso in correct neutral pelvis/neutral spine shows the ribcage relaxed and low to the ground.

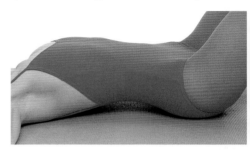

Here the torso is in incorrect neutral pelvis/neutral spine alignment. Notice that the waist is too high off the floor, tipping the pelvis and causing the back to arch upwards.

lying on your back

Lie on your back with your feet parallel and flat on the floor, and hip-width apart. Point your toes forwards. The knees should be bent and hip-width apart, and the hips and tailbone are on the floor, but the waist is slightly off the floor at the curve of the lower back. The back of the ribcage touches the floor, but the back of the neck curve does not. Remember, the spine is long in this position but it still has its two natural curves that do not touch the floor – at the lower back and at the neck.

The shoulders are down on the floor, the neck is long, and the front of the throat is relaxed. Resting your head on a thin pillow, find a position for it that lets your throat stay soft, and stops your chin pulling down onto the chest or backwards. Your arms are at your sides, the elbows softly bent and pointing outwards, and your palms to the floor.

It is most important that the back of the ribcage is supported by the floor. You may find that you can't have your back touching and still have your tailbone touching

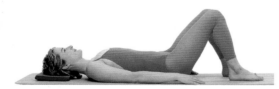

Find neutral pelvis/neutral spine alignment by lying on your back with your knees bent and feet flat on the floor – both hip-width apart. The spine is flat to the floor except for the curve of the lower back and the back of the neck.

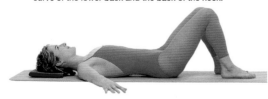

Notice as you lie in this position that the back of your ribcage is touching the floor, but the curve of your lower back is slightly off the floor, but without arching.

with your pelvis in neutral. Keeping the spine supported by the floor should be your priority. In time, as you gain more experience, your spine will lengthen and you'll find this easier. Neutral pelvis means that your pubic bone, hips and belly button are on a flat plane parallel to the floor. Try not to have your pubic bone higher than your navel.

This exercise will help you to find neutral pelvis/neutral spine quickly and easily. As you lie on your back in the position described above, tip your pelvis North (pressing your waist back onto the floor), losing the curve in your lower back. Now tip in the opposite direction so that your lower back overarches as your waist lifts away from the floor – overarching too much may not feel pleasant! Then find the midpoint between these two extremes. This is neutral. You can slip one hand under your waist and feel a slight gap between your waist and the floor. You should be able to find this neutral pelvis/neutral spine starting position when you are standing or sitting, or lying on your back, side or stomach, or kneeling on all fours. Your pelvis should also be level from East to West, so do not allow your hips to tip to the right or left. Keep the front of the ribcage soft: do not let the ribs flare out.

lying face-down

Lie on your stomach, and rest your forehead lightly on the floor. Your arms are extended in front of you, palms to the floor. The neck is long, and the shoulders and upper back are open, relaxed and down. Keep your spine long. Your ribcage, pubic bone and hip bones touch the floor, but your navel hovers just above it. Your stomach flesh may touch the floor, but don't push your stomach into the floor as that will tighten up your lower back and shorten it. Your legs are hip-width apart. Practise to get this right!

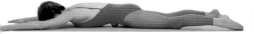

A ball under your navel lets you feel how the abdominals lift.

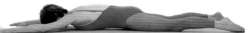

Now take the ball away and try to keep the abdominals lifted.

lying on your side

Lie on your side in a straight line from head to toes. To do this, line your body up with the back edge of the mat, with one hip bone stacked directly on top of the other, and one shoulder directly over the other, and your spine long. The waist does not touch the floor. Your bottom arm is extended straight up above your head and your elbow then bends and your hand rests on the back of your head to support your head and neck. Bring your feet slightly forward until the toes are just about reaching the front edge of the mat. Even though you appear to be lying in a straight line you still maintain your natural curves, at your lower back and the back of the neck.

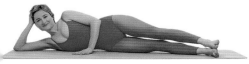

Notice how the waist is off the floor and hip is over hip.

on hands and knees

Kneel on your hands and knees, with your hands directly below your shoulders and your knees right below your hips, hip-width apart. The pelvis and the spine are in neutral. To find this, tip your pelvis so that the pubic bone comes towards your chest, then tip it again so that the pubic bone pushes away from the chest. In this small movement you will find the curve in your lower back increases or decreases. Neutral pelvis will be the point between the two extremes. The neck is long and in line with the spine, the chin tips slightly towards the chest, and you look at the floor. Lift your breastbone/chest upwards so that the area on your upper back between the shoulder blades is raised and not hollow.

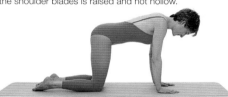

The spine is long and the neck stays in line with the spine.

sitting

Sit upright with your weight evenly distributed on both buttocks. The spine and neck are long, the chin is parallel to the floor, and the shoulder blades pulled down towards the waist. Your breastbone lifts softly upwards and the chest is open. Check the position of your head in relation to your shoulders and hips. Your navel is back to your spine, the natural curves at your waist and at the back of the neck still present. The knees and parallel feet are hip-width apart, feet flat on the floor.

The head is placed directly over the shoulders and hips in line.

Engaging the pelvic floor

In each exercise you will hear me say 'engage the pelvic floor', 'draw your navel back to your spine', or 'hollow your stomach'. This all translates as 'strongly engage your deep stomach muscles'! In pilates we engage below the tummy area so that we have full, free breathing without squeezing the ribcage together – which would restrict our breathing and not allow us to take in maximum oxygen. So we engage in the pelvic floor, which runs from the anal opening to the front genitals on the underside of the body between the legs. The pelvic floor can be engaged by contracting any of its muscular openings. Women have three openings they can choose to engage: the vaginal muscles, the anal muscles and the urethra muscles, which feel as though you are stopping the flow of urine when you engage. Men have just two: the anal and the urethra muscles. Practise engaging these muscles without moving your pelvis while you are lying on your back in your alignment position, the relaxation pose, with a neutral pelvis and a neutral spine.

When we engage the pelvic floor muscles we also trigger the deepest of the abdominal muscles, the transversus abdominus, which is a very important muscle for maintaining good upright posture. The transversus starts at the pubic bone and runs up to the breastbone then wraps around the waist and supports the lower back. We call this the 'girdle of strength', and if you can strengthen your transversus, you will before long notice a huge improvement in your posture and in your performance of all the pilates exercises.

testing the pelvic floor muscles

To test if you are engaging the pelvic floor correctly, simply press the first two fingers of both hands down on the area just above your pubic bone as you engage either the vaginal, anal or urethra muscles. If you have engaged properly you will probably feel a slight movement under your fingertips. Practise engaging the pelvic floor on an exhaled breath, and releasing on an inhaled breath, for five breaths. Then engage the pelvic floor and hold that engagement for five breaths.

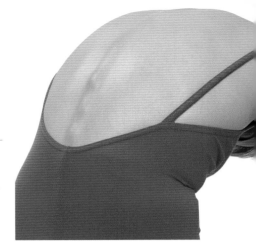

The spine is round, not flat, and rolls like a wheel.

Articulating the spine

You will come across this term in this book. It refers to movement in the spine where we individually move one vertebra at a time and feel the movement from the bottom to the top of the spine or from top to bottom. The spine has 24 moving vertebrae and each vertebra, if healthy, is a joint with movement for bending forward, bending backwards, bending sideways to left or right and rotating round to the left or to the right. You may feel that there are sections in your spine which resist movement. Breathe deeply in these areas and focus on a little more movement each time to free up your spine.

Chin to chest

This term refers to the placement of the head in relation to the spine. When an exercise calls for you to put your chin to your chest, you rotate your head downwards from the jawbone. The rotation should be in the jaw joint as you tip your chin down. The head then comes forward above the breastbone to leave a space between the chin and the chest, your eyes fixing on your pubic bone. Do not pull your chin and strain the front of the throat. The position of the head is very important because the weight of the head drawn forwards both decreases neck tension and increases work in the deep abdominals. It may be difficult at first to bring your chin to your chest, as your deep abdominals may be quite weak. Do only as many repetitions as you can without pain or strain.

Lateral breathing

In pilates we have a very specific style of breathing. We inhale through the nose and exhale through the mouth. As we inhale, the ribcage expands wide out to the sides, and as we exhale, the ribcage closes down, like a pair of bellows. Throughout most of the day we are probably only taking short shallow breaths and not even expanding the lower lungs, so it may be a bit difficult at first.

Imagine as you inhale that the breath comes into you like water, pouring down into the lowest part of the lungs first (which is the waist area); and then, as you exhale, that the water is being poured out, the air leaving the uppermost part of the lungs first and the lower lungs last. Because the filling lungs are beneath the ribs, the ribcage expands as you inhale. The lungs empty and get smaller as you exhale, of course, and the ribcage shrinks.

breathing with a band
We can practise a lateral breathing exercise sitting down, lying on our backs or kneeling in an upright position.

Wrap a stretchy rubber exercise band or towel around the widest part of your ribcage. With each hand holding one end of the band, cross the band at the front of the ribcage. As you inhale into the deep lungs, the ribcage expands and you loosen the band slightly to allow this to happen. When you exhale, the lungs empty and the ribcage becomes smaller so you tighten the rubber band to help reinforce this. You will notice that the ribcage is actually expanding sideways and contracting with each inhale and exhale. Try not to lift the chest, arms or shoulders as you breathe. Watch yourself in a mirror for a few times and see what happens. As we breathe in this way we can exercise, engaging the pelvic floor for strength and stability in the body without stopping the ribcage movements. If you push your stomach out during each inhale, you will not be able to engage the deep abdominals correctly, so please try to master this technique for the best development of those deep core stabilizing muscles! Inhale for about five seconds and exhale for about five seconds, if that is comfortable for you. Avoid holding your breath for difficult movements: this can cause tension and can strain the heart.

equipment

Yoga mat A sticky rectangular rubber mat measuring about 180 x 60 cm (72 x 24 in) and about 4–6 mm (⅙–¼ in) thick. Yoga mats protect the spine and prevent slipping. They are available in shops and on the internet.

Blankets Single-size blanket made of wool or cotton, approximately 150 x 200 cm (62 x 80 in). The blanket, folded several times into a rectangle, provides a firm raised surface for you to sit on or lie over. You can also roll three blankets together to make a higher surface, like a bolster.

Bolster A specially designed firm cylindrical pillow available from yoga supply firms. The bolster provides a firm rounded surface to lie over.

Yoga block A block of foam which provides a raised surface for support for hands, fingers, feet or hips.

Yoga brick A brick-shaped prop made of foam, wood or cork which supports hands, fingers, feet or hips.

Yoga belt/strap A custom-design cotton belt with a buckle about 1.6 m (6 ft) long . The belt generally allows you to reach some part of your body, such as the toes that you are normally unable to reach. If you don't have one, try a bathrobe belt or any other cloth belt.

Bands Stretchy bands in various thicknesses of latex rubber which provide resistance or support.

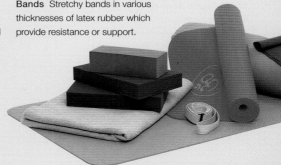

meditation techniques

et's begin… connect with yourself. Meditation is the magic that brings you into yourself and gives you time just to observe yourself and be in the moment. Forget the past, forget the future – can you really just be here, now? Meditation has so many benefits. Most people start meditating to calm themselves and feel better, more relaxed. As you begin, you will soon realize how amazing meditation is and you will want to go even further. Not only will you feel calmer, you will probably also notice how much clearer your thoughts are. You can sit down to meditate and afterwards come up with answers to questions you hadn't even asked. Your mind becomes more creative when you are 'connected' with yourself. You will process everything much more quickly. You may notice that you suddenly find the rest of the world is very slow as you calmly move at a faster and faster pace. This doesn't mean that you start running around instead of walking, just that you can think about something and then quickly process it, make decisions and manifest it. Clarity becomes more and more noticeable as you become more experienced in meditation. You become more observant, more empowered, more focused and clearer, and then, with less effort than before, more creative. You may also notice that you feel better physically: as you get more relaxed in yourself, your muscles will start to relax too.

We all know of the amazing influence the mind has on the body and when we are calm, healthy and strong in our mind it should follow that we are also relaxed, healthy and strong in our bodies. This was the purpose of meditation and yoga. To begin meditating I'll introduce you to a

Sitting on a cushion or foam block during breathing and meditation exercises helps to lift the spine upwards in correct alignment.

simple yet very effective meditation technique. Practise with this one technique initially, and when you feel comfortable with your meditation practice you may want to expand your repertoire by reading about other techniques or attending a class.

Here are a few suggestions for meditating:
- Try to establish a regular time and place, especially when you are first starting out. When you wake up in the morning and just before bedtime are usually good choices for a few minutes of meditation.
- Choose a special place to meditate, somewhere peaceful and quiet, beautiful and inspiring. You may want to build a little altar, with flowers or special items that you value. Try to settle in that place every day, to start with, if this is possible.
- Find a comfortable position to sit in. You do not have to sit cross-legged on the floor in agony! It is important that you keep your spine straight and the front of your body open, not collapsed forward. For easy breathing to occur, the ribcage must be open. You can sit in a straight-backed chair, keeping your spine straight and your feet on the floor, or you can sit cross-legged against a wall to support the spine. Or sit on a block or a meditation cushion, which is just a few centimetres high, to lift your hips higher off the floor so sitting is more comfortable and it's easier to keep your spine straight. If you sit in a position which is not comfortable to start with, your mind will be distracted by the pain and meditation will feel strained.
- When you are first starting out it is quite beneficial to be in a quiet room. When you are more experienced you will find that you can block out noise and meditate anywhere, but at first noise may distract you.

Breathing and focusing

So now you are sitting comfortably in a quiet place at your chosen time. Forget the past, forget the future: be here, now. Command the mind to still. To help this, have a few minutes of deep breathing. You will inhale through your nose and exhale through your nose. This is more efficient breathing for this practice and will stimulate more nerve endings than breathing through your mouth, helping to relax you. As you inhale, count to five seconds, and as you exhale, count to five seconds. When this becomes easy increase the time to maybe ten seconds. This builds up strength in the lungs and diaphragm and settles the mind, slowing it down. After a few minutes of this breathing technique you should feel still and ready to meditate. Allow your breathing to become regular. Do not concentrate so much on breathing correctly that you become stressed – just continue to breathe with your mouth closed, inhaling and exhaling through your nose in a relaxed way. Allow your mind to still. Watch the breath as it enters and leaves your nostrils. Settle into the rhythm.

Focus on the point between the eyebrows, which is an important energy centre in the body. Bringing your attention here is said to stimulate nerve endings which release chemicals in the body to make you feel good! Now observe the feeling in that area between the eyebrows. How does it feel? Is there a pulse there? Do you feel a heavy throb, or is the area light and tingly? Just observe this single point and you will be accomplishing what we call single-point focus, which teaches the mind to concentrate on one thing at a time and not be distracted. Do not allow other thoughts to interrupt your observation. If they do come into your head, allow them to leave without getting angry or frustrated about this 'failure' in your concentration. Learning not to become attached to the results of your actions is part of the

The front of the body is long and open and the chest and shoulders are relaxed.

goal of meditation, so start in a small way here. Enjoy the experience and the new things you will observe and learn, and don't always look for a particular goal.

Now shift the focus to another body part near the last one, such as the tip of your nose. Stay there for a few minutes and observe the feelings. Then move on again – to the top and bottom lips, the chin, the neck, the throat, the chest, the arms, hands, fingers and so on, until you have worked around the entire body. This will give you something to focus on that requires no thought or imagination, just observation of something tangible, our own body, which we know to be true. If we meditate on a particular word or image the mind is often still active and will not settle as it is busy with imagery and reactions to scenarios being created in the mind. Meditation is not a trance either. We want to be able to hear the things in the room, as if we are aware of our surroundings but not distracted or anxious about them. This supports the purpose of meditation in training the mind to find single-point focus, keeping the mind still, and remaining aware of what is happening around us without disturbing ourselves.

Can you just be here, right now, and let your mind become so quiet that you can feel the blood pumping through your body? See if you can feel and hear the pulse in your solar plexus area, just below the breastbone and above the navel. The corners of the mouth may begin to turn up slightly with no effort and you may feel yourself sway slightly. Don't worry if this happens. You may also observe colours. There is no way to explain the bliss that you feel when you are connected with yourself in meditation. You will have to experience it for yourself as it is different for everyone. Try to meditate for five minutes at a time to start with, working up to about 20 minutes if you can. Don't be frustrated if your concentration is broken with the occasional thought passing through. You will still have those precious moments of uninterrupted bliss! After your meditation session we will move on to a very simple breathing exercise – to oxygenate the blood, calm the mind and also to strengthen the lungs and all the muscles associated with breathing. The list of benefits from deep breathing is huge: all the cells of your body will benefit. More than anything, the body needs the basics of water and air, so you will feel and look better if you practise regular deep-breathing exercises such as this.

Pranayama breathing

Pranayama is a yogic breathing exercise said to control the energy. In yoga the breath is seen as energy. Learning to control it is said to teach us how to control our energy. Sit in a comfortable position. We will continue to use closed-mouth breathing, so remember to inhale and exhale through the nose. Breathing should be even at the beginning and at the end of each breath so you will have to learn to control the breath rather than taking it all in quickly, or just getting rid of it all at once.

To start with, try counting to five seconds for the inhale and five for the exhale. Do not strain to meet this breathing cycle. If five is too long, then change it to maybe three seconds. The breath is very directly connected to the nervous system and the benefits of the breathing exercise will be lost if you are straining just to achieve a goal. Breathe in a range that suits you and does not create anxiety. Progress will inevitably take time, but will happen, so there is no need to push yourself to the point

of stress and tension. Take two easy full breaths before you begin the exercise and then, on the third breath, inhale until your lungs are about halfway full and then hold the breath for five seconds. Release for five seconds then inhale fully for five seconds; then exhale fully for five seconds. Inhale fully for five seconds, exhale fully for five seconds, then inhale only halfway full and hold the breath for five seconds. Exhale fully for five seconds. Then repeat this cycle of two normal full breaths and then holding the breath for five seconds – five times if it's comfortable. This gives you a taste of a new strong breathing technique and will provide some nice benefits!

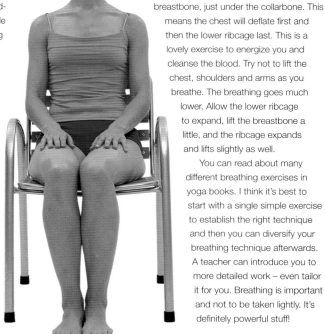

As you inhale, imagine the breath travelling to the lowest past of your lungs at the bottom of the ribcage at your waist. This means the lower ribcage will expand first and then the chest. As you exhale, imagine the breath flowing out from the highest point of the lungs, the area above the breastbone, just under the collarbone. This means the chest will deflate first and then the lower ribcage last. This is a lovely exercise to energize you and cleanse the blood. Try not to lift the chest, shoulders and arms as you breathe. The breathing goes much lower. Allow the lower ribcage to expand, lift the breastbone a little, and the ribcage expands and lifts slightly as well.

You can read about many different breathing exercises in yoga books. I think it's best to start with a single simple exercise to establish the right technique and then you can diversify your breathing technique afterwards. A teacher can introduce you to more detailed work – even tailor it for you. Breathing is important and not to be taken lightly. It's definitely powerful stuff!

understanding the spine

The first structure formed in a child's body in the mother's womb is the spine. All other limbs develop from it, so the spine is very important. All movement should come from the spine, so a stable, strong spine is a stable base for all actions. A baby's spine is soft and light, and it remains so for a long time, whereas an adult spine is usually heavy and rigid.

Using the programme in this book we will try to develop correct movement patterns, break bad habits and return the spine to its former suppleness. A baby's spine is straight until the baby begins to walk, when it develops curves that it will keep for the rest of its life. These curves are developed as shock absorbers. An animal or a baby has a straight spine while it is on four legs, but when the body is upright, on two legs, the spine cannot be straight as too much pressure would be placed on the soft discs sitting between each vertebra. The spine should have three natural curves: in the cervical spine at the back of the neck; in the thoracic spine at the back of the ribcage; and in the lower back, known as the lumbar spine (see diagram, right). The curves can be lesser or greater than they should be for a healthy spine, due to bad posture, a particular habit or sport that develops the muscles of the body in an uneven way, or through an injury, among various other possible reasons.

The cervical spine has 7 cervical vertebrae, the thoracic spine has 12 thoracic vertebrae and the lumbar spine has 5 lumbar vertebrae, all with soft discs between each vertebra. The spine is not a stiff, straight piece of bone, but a collection of 24 separate movable vertebrae made of bone, connected by several layers of muscles that crisscross like shoe laces, from vertebra to vertebra, up and down the spine to hold it together. The thoracic spine also has connecting ribs, making this area a bit less flexible than other parts of the spine. Each vertebra can move forwards, backwards and sideways to the left and right, and can also rotate, to the left or right. Because the head is supported by the spine, which is supported by the pelvis, which is supported by the legs, which are, in turn, supported by the feet, lining up all these elements is crucial for a healthy, pain-free spine.

Over the years general wear and tear on the discs or bad posture may result in damage to a disc and accompanying pain. By learning a little about the spine and a lot about good posture and good movement patterns, this may be avoided. If you have back pain or an injury now, or have had in the past, please see your doctor before starting this – or any – exercise programme, or you may aggravate the problem. It's good to see if your doctor recommends the exercises and, if not, what might be permissible. For example, if you have injured a disc, then bending forward will irritate the injury and cause great pain. The spine is a hard-working collection of fascinating parts, which all deserve your respect. Please listen to your body and if you are in pain, see a doctor. You may find that a pain-free spine is still possible.

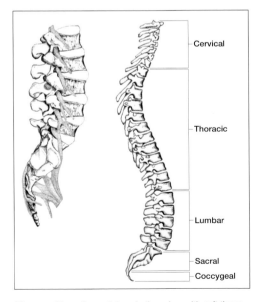

There are 24 moving vertebrae in the spine, with soft tissue discs between each vertebra. Note the curves in the spine.

pre-exercise

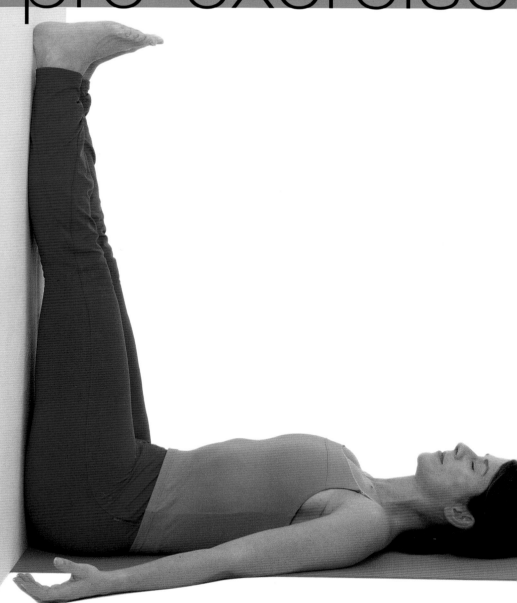

& warm-up

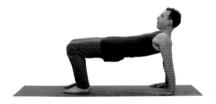

Make sure you read 'getting started' (see pages 12–23) and practise the breathing, alignment and pelvic-floor engagement exercises described there before you begin the six 'pre-exercises' in this chapter – designed for people who are either new to movement or recovering from injury, or perhaps just not ready emotionally for a challenging workout. Limit yourself to the pre-exercise programme until you feel that you can complete it easily, without feeling breathless or dizzy. And then progress to the three-exercise warm-up sequence (see pages 34–7) which you should do immediately before both the beginner's and intermediate programmes too.

For more details on this exercise, see pages 34–5.

samasthiti to mountain pose

aims

to lengthen the spine and the neck; to link the body and the mind through breath; to build awareness of posture; to open and strengthen the shoulder joints; and to stretch the arms, hands and fingers.

1 Stand in correct alignment with your feet very close together, touching if you feel stable enough. Press your feet down into the floor, keep your legs straight without locking your knees, while your spine lifts up to the sky. Without arching the back or pushing out the ribcage in front of you, lift your chest. Now lengthen your neck by lifting your head upwards, with your chin parallel to the floor and your shoulder blades gently moving down. Keep your arms straight and open at the elbows, wrists and palms, with your fingertips pointing downwards.

2 Inhale, sweep your arms up from each side towards your head. Keep your palms facing downwards until you reach the halfway point.

3 Then spin your palms to face up as you finish the move by bringing your palms together in prayer, hands above your head, as you gaze up at your hands. Lean backwards slightly, keeping your chest lifted and your tailbone slightly tucked under. As you reach up, drop your ribcage down. Keep your arms straight with your palms facing each other or with your hands just touching if that is more comfortable. Exhale, then reverse the sequence and take your arms back down to your starting position. Repeat four times.

reminders: Here, strong breath links body and mind. Remember to keep your hips stable and to lengthen your spine.

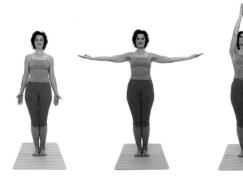

chiropractor's comments

Excellent for making you aware of your spine and posture. Keep your neck long and relaxed as you pull your shoulder blades down. Feel the activation of the muscles in your middle back.

marching on the spot

aims

improves coordination between left and right sides; develops flexibility in the hip and knee; strengthens the hip flexor muscles; develops core strength; and provides cardio work.

1   Start in good standing alignment, with your feet hip-width apart.

2   Lift one knee as high as is comfortable and then lower it and repeat on the other side. Keep correct alignment with a long spine and your arms relaxed. March at a good pace for about 25 seconds.

3   Now crisscross your arms towards your opposite knees as you march, while keeping your spine upright and correct alignment. The knees and elbows don't meet. Breathe fully, counting to about five seconds each time you inhale and for another five on each exhalation.

reminders: Maintain good alignment by standing tall. Don't fold your body forward towards your knees. Look straight ahead at all times and keep your navel pulled in to your spine, while your chest is lifted high.

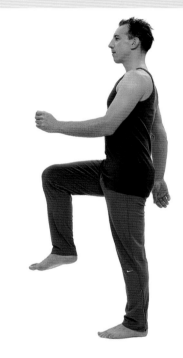

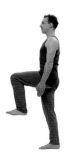
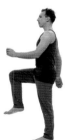

arm circles

aims

to open and strengthen the rotator cuff muscles of the shoulder joints; to stabilize the shoulders, and restore full range of movement in the shoulder joints; to improve circulation to the upper body; and to build core strength.

1 Stand in good alignment, with your feet slightly apart and pointing forwards and your arms and hands loosely at each side.

2 Raise your arms out sideways to just below shoulder level, slightly in front of the body. Stand tall, lift your chest and drop your shoulder blades. Pull through the middle finger of each hand to lengthen your arms away from your shoulders.

3 Start to make small circles with your arms, keeping your shoulder blades down as you circle and pulling your arms away from your shoulders to lengthen them. Keep your chest lifted and your neck long. Now increase the size of the circles, focusing even more on holding your shoulder blades down as you lengthen and straighten your arms. Breathe deeply, inhaling for five counts, exhaling for five counts; this will provide enough oxygen to work the muscles without exhausting you, forcing you to give up!

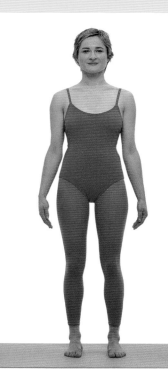

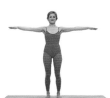
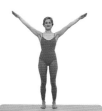

4 Increase the size of the circles even more so that your fingertips point up to the sky or down to the ground at the highest and lowest points, remembering to focus on keeping your shoulder blades down as you do so. At this point your breathing has to be even deeper to keep your arms travelling at the same rate, and not allowing one side to become dominant. Now reverse the direction of the circles and reverse all your actions. Do 30 circles in each direction.

chiropractor's comments
Keep your shoulder joints level with each other; do not let one side lift higher than the other with the movement. Keep squared and strong in your abdominal and pelvic muscles.

reminders: Make sure you keep your chest open and lifted and your shoulders down, away from your ears. Remember to engage your abdominals tightly throughout.

relaxation pose to backstroke/starfish

aims

to establish good alignment and good movement patterns throughout the body; and to maintain a strong centre while moving; to lengthen the spine and improve coordination.

1 Assume a neutral pelvis/neutral spine starting position as you lie on your back with a thin pillow beneath your head. Your arms should be on the floor at your sides, your palms facing down and your elbows softly bent out to each side. Your knees are bent, and your knees and feet are hip-width apart. Your spine should be on the mat – except at its natural curves – and the back of your ribcage should stay in contact with the floor.

2 Inhale to prepare. Exhale, engage your pelvic floor and draw your navel back to your spine, keeping alignment. Don't tip your pelvis. Lift your right arm to the ceiling, and then backwards – without actually touching the floor behind your head. Keep your ribcage on the floor and lengthen your spine.

3 Inhale and bring your right arm back up to the vertical, with your fingertips reaching up towards the ceiling. As you do this, bring your left arm up to same point, so that both your arms are straight above your chest, shoulder-width apart, with your palms facing your feet. Keep the alignment throughout.

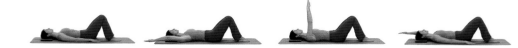

4 Exhale. Now take your left arm back behind you and move your right arm forward in the opposite direction. Maintain alignment, remembering to keep the back of the ribcage down. The arms are soft, yet long. Don't lock your elbows, and keep your shoulder blades down. The front of the ribcage stays low. Reverse and repeat the arm sequence five times.

5 Now return to the neutral starting position. Recheck the alignment, focusing on keeping the navel, public bone and hip bones on a plane. When you are ready inhale, then exhale, and engage the pelvic floor.

6 Slide your left leg along the floor away from the hips as you take the right arm above and behind you in a backstroke movement. maintain neutral pelvis/neutral spine and keep your shoulder blades down. Inhale and return both the arm and leg to the starting position simultaneously.

7 Exhale. Then take your left arm backwards and your right arm forwards, maintaining alignment. Don't lock your elbows; the arms should be soft but long. Move your shoulder blades away from your ears, down towards your waist. Keep the front of your ribcage low. Reverse and repeat the whole sequence a further four times.

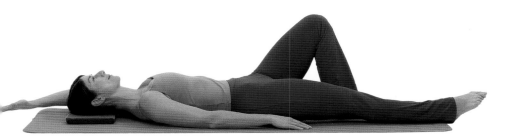

chiropractor's comments

An important exercise for unstable low backs. Maintain stability and control during the arm and leg movements. Keep your awareness on your lower back to prevent any overarching of your lower spine!

reminders: Concentration is required here! This seems easy, but it is hard to do it properly. Keep the back of your ribcage down on the floor and your shoulder blades down.

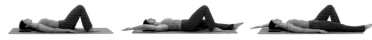

seated wide-angle pose

aims

to stretch the spine, sides of trunk, inner thighs and hamstrings while stabilizing in a correct alignment. Opens the rotator cuff muscles in the shoulders and stabilizes the shoulder joints.

chiropractor's comments

A great exercise for feeling the symmetrical motion of the shoulders, while maintaining a neutral pelvis and spine. Be careful – do not overarch your lower spine.

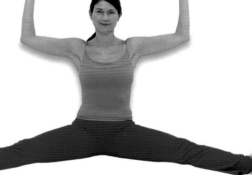

1 Sit on the floor with your back and hips against a wall, legs straight out in front of you. Sit on a pillow (or phone directory) to avoid rounding your lower back. Now draw your legs apart so that your knees and toes point to the sky and the backs of your knees are to the floor. Lift yourself onto your hands, positioned on either side of your hips, raising your pelvis off the floor briefly. Then sit down again – flat on your sitting bones, with your buttocks on the floor. Your lower back is long and lifted, your neck is long, and the back of your ribcage should touch the wall.

2 Inhale, and raise both arms up along the wall in a circular movement, keeping your shoulder blades down and your ribcage against the wall.

3 Bring your arms up higher until your hands almost meet above your head to complete the circle. Maintain your alignment, and keep your arms and hands in continuous contact with the wall.

4 Exhale then reverse the movement, taking the arms back down to the starting position. Repeat the exercise five times.

reminders: Sit up tall, keep your shoulder blades down and lift your breastbone. Keep the front of your ribcage wide open, not closed in or collapsed. The navel is back towards the spine so the pelvis is not tilted and the tailbone points down towards the floor.

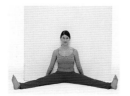
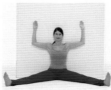
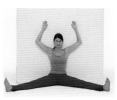
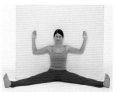

legs up the wall

aims

to improve concentration and stretch the spine and hamstrings; to remove fatigue; and to relieve varicose veins. The downward flow of blood cleanses the lower limbs and nourishes the upper body, neck and head.

chiropractor's comments

This is an excellent way to stretch your gluteal muscles and hamstrings. Please proceed with caution, though, and ask your doctor's advice if you have a history of disc-related problems.

1 Lie with your right side down on the floor, with your knees tucked to your chest and your buttocks against the wall.

2 Carefully turn over so that your back is flat on the floor and your tailbone is touching the wall. Keep your hips square and your head pointing away from the wall. Slowly extend one leg up the wall.

3 Now extend the other leg up the wall, so that both legs are straight and the backs of the legs are against the wall. Lie flat on the floor with your arms straight but easy, just away from your body, palms facing upwards. Breathe comfortably and remain in this pose for one to three minutes. Then come down by slowly bending your knees and rolling onto your side.

reminders: If you find this uncomfortable, take your hips further away from the wall.

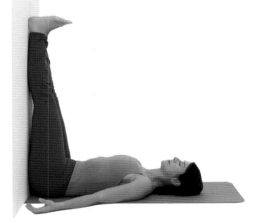

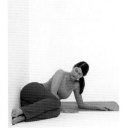
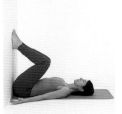
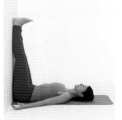

samasthiti to mountain pose

aims

to lengthen the spine and the neck; to link the body and mind through breath; to build awareness of posture; to open and strengthen the shoulder joints; and to stretch the arms, hands and fingers.

1 Stand in correct alignment with your feet very close together; they could be touching if you feel stable enough. Press your feet down into the floor, keep your legs straight without locking your knees back and lift your spine up to the sky.

Without arching your back or pushing your ribcage out in front, lift your chest. Lengthen the neck as your head lifts upwards in order to keep your chin parallel to the floor, and gently move your shoulder blades down.

Keep your arms straight and open at the elbows, so that your wrists and palms are facing towards the front and your fingertips are extended softly downwards towards the floor.

2 Inhale. Sweep your arms up from your sides towards your head. Keep your palms facing downwards until you reach the halfway point.

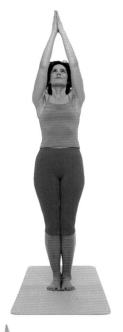

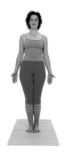
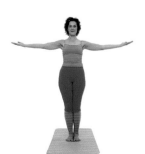
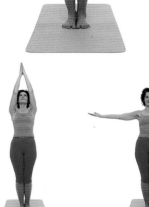

3 Now spin your palms to face upwards as you finish the move, bringing your palms together in prayer hands above your head, and gazing up at your hands. Lean backwards slightly, keeping your chest lifted and your tailbone slightly tucked under. As you reach up, drop your ribcage down and keep your arms straight with your palms facing each other or even touching, if you feel comfortable enough.

4 Exhale, and take your arms back down to the sides, with your palms facing up until they reach shoulder height.

5 Now return to your starting position. Then you should repeat the whole opening, stretching sequence a further four times.

reminders: Strong breathing links the body and the mind here. Keep your hips stable and your spine long.

---

chiropractor's comments
Keep your pelvic muscles actively engaged, visualize and feel your stomach muscles holding tight while the lower back is lifting. Feel your spine becoming longer!

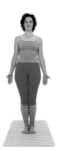

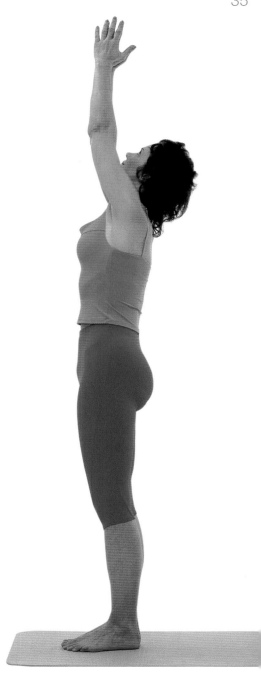

chicken wings on the wall

aims

to strengthen, stabilize and open the shoulder joints; to practise correct alignment against a wall, where we can easily check our own alignment; to build core stability.

1 Stand in correct alignment against a wall, with your feet, hip-width apart, about 30 cm (12 in) away from it. Lean back so that your hips touch the wall and your back is supported. Keep the legs long, but your knees softly bent. Rest your head against the wall with your chin parallel to the floor. The arms are out at shoulder height, with the elbows at an angle of 90 degrees against the wall – palms to the front and fingertips upwards.

2 Inhale to prepare, then exhale. Engage your pelvic floor as you slide your arms about 12.5 cm (5 in) higher up the wall. Keep the back of your ribcage against the wall and don't arch your back.

3 Inhale, and slide your arms down the wall to just below your start position, trying to keep the hands, arms and the back of the ribcage in contact with it. Exhale, and repeat five times.

reminders: Your arms, hands and the back of the ribcage are in constant contact with the wall.

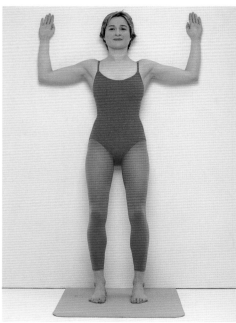

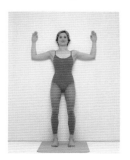
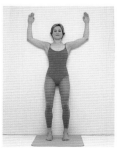
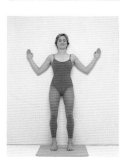

chiropractor's comments

Great for building stability in the lower spine. Targets pelvic and spinal muscles, while working on the range of motion of your shoulder blades.

the chair

aims

to learn correct alignment; to lengthen the base of the spine; and to correct the pelvis-to-spine angle. Builds deep abdominal strength and strength in the thighs and buttocks; and stretches the Achilles tendon.

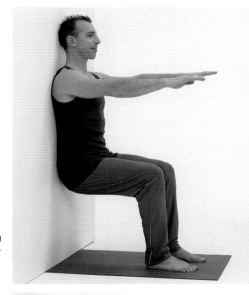

1   Stand against the wall in correct alignment and take your feet forwards about 45 cm (18 in). Place your feet hip-width apart, parallel to each other and lean back so that your spine and head touch the wall. Allow space for the curves in the lower back and at the back of the neck. Raise your arms in front of you, parallel to the floor – palms down.

2   Inhale, bend your knees and slide down the wall until your thighs are parallel to the floor. Keep your heels flat and your knees over your feet. Your spine stays in contact with the wall.

3   Exhale, engage pelvic floor and deep abdominals and slide back up, keeping your spine and head in contact with the wall, your arms parallel to the floor and your spine long. Inhale and repeat five times.

reminders: At the lowest point of the bend your knees should be directly over your midfoot, forming a right angle between the thighs and calves. Your head and shoulders stay on the wall throughout. Keep your shoulders down, away from your ears.

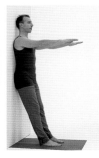
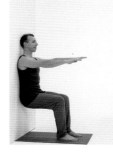
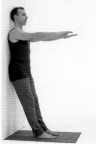

chiropractor's comments
Exercises and strengthens the anterior thigh muscles (quadriceps) while maintaining a strong neutral pelvis.

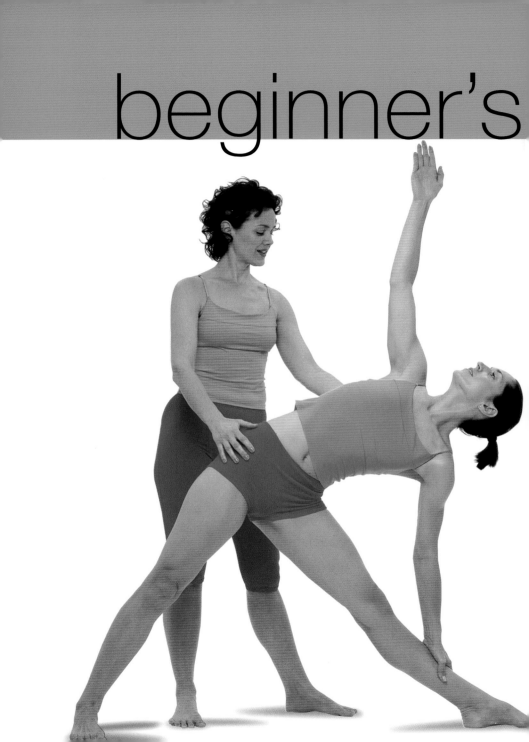

beginner's

programme

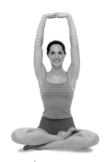

The beginner's programme teaches you how to work from a strong centre. Before you attempt it, please read 'getting started' (see pages 12–23), making sure that you are able to engage the pelvic floor, perform lateral breathing in the ribcage and locate correct neutral pelvis/neutral spine alignment whether you are standing, kneeling or lying. Please make sure you do the three warm-up exercises (see pages 34–7) before you start, too. Then you should work with the programme until you know that you can complete the twenty exercises in an easy, relaxed manner, breathing comfortably and with no pain. Only when you can do this will you be ready for the challenges of the intermediate programme.

roll down on the wall

aims

to relax the spine, increasing the space between each vertebra, allowing the discs to expand and the spine to lengthen; to relax the shoulders and chest; to create flexibility and strength in the spine. Also teaches spinal articulation, strengthens the abdominals and builds core strength.

1 Stand about 30 cm (12 in) away from the wall, with your feet parallel and hip-width apart and your knees hip-width apart. Lean back on the wall to support your spine. The knees are softly bent so that you are comfortable and in correct alignment, keeping the pelvis neutral. Inhale and lengthen through the spine.

2 Exhale, and then begin to peel your spine off the wall. Softly drop your chin towards your chest as you release your head and neck, and let the weight of your head draw you down towards the floor. Roll through your spine as if it were a wheel, one vertebra at a time. Feel each vertebra touch the wall before it peels off.

3 As you roll lower, let your arms dangle like the arms of a puppet, without any tension, and lift the navel higher towards the spine so that the front of your body feels lifted, helping to open the back of the body.

chiropractor's comments
A great warm-up for your spine! Proceed slowly and try to become aware of the individual segmental movement that can occur in your upper–lower back. Feel the gentle mobilization of the spine – its flexibility and strength. Because it involves forward flexion of the lumbar spine, you should consult your doctor if you have a history of lower back or disc-related injury.

4 When you have rolled down completely, inhale, and then exhale, reversing the downward roll to come back up to a standing position. Press one vertebra at a time back into the wall as you roll up, dropping your tailbone down.

5 Your head, neck and shoulders are the last to come up. Stand in correct alignment and take a few deep breaths. Repeat the roll down and roll back up sequence five times.

reminders: Try to roll down in centre and avoid swaying from side to side. Make sure that your weight is evenly distributed on both feet.

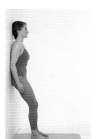
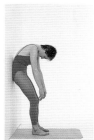
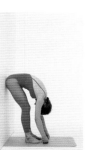
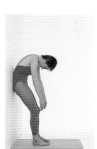
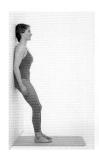

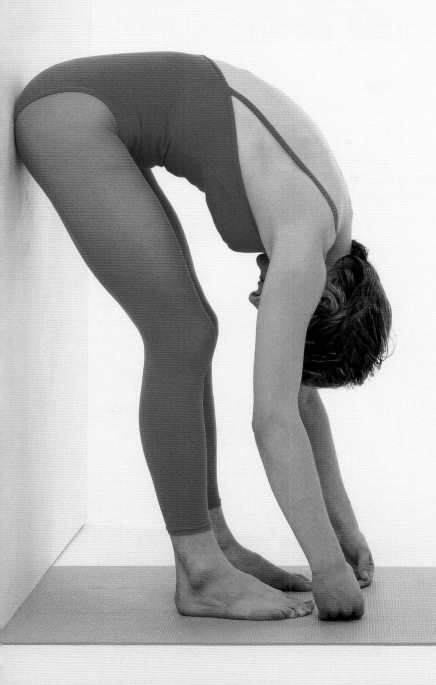

L-shape pelvic tilt

aims

to lengthen the hamstrings; to develop awareness, strength and flexibility in the lower back; and to release any tension in the shoulders and upper back.

1 Stand facing a tabletop. Place your hands on the table at about hip height, shoulder-width apart. Step back from the support until your feet are directly under your hips. Lean forwards as you stretch out your spine, and press your hands into the tabletop. Inhale and lift the buttocks towards the ceiling to stretch the back of the legs. Feel your spine lengthen. Expand the chest, open the armpits and broaden the upper back. Exhale, tuck your pelvis under slightly, and bring the pubic

chiropractor's comments

Activates and stretches the hamstrings, mainly felt at their pelvic attachment. Relax through the upper back and feel the stretch around your shoulders. This allows movement to occur between the segmental joints of the spine. Use caution if you suffer from lower back or shoulder problems.

bone up towards the chest to stretch the lower back. Tip your pelvis back and forth several times, breathing with the rhythm of this movement.

reminders: Small movement equals big stretch. This action should feel as though it takes place below the waist. Keep lengthening the upper body as you gently tip your pelvis back and forth.

tennis ball lift

aims

to build strong alignment of the feet, ankles, knees and hips; and to strengthen the front of the thighs, stabilizing the muscles of the knee.

1 Stand in correct alignment. Place a tennis ball between your ankles, just below the ankle bone. Inhale, lengthen up through the spine and hold your tailbone down.

2 Exhale. Pull your navel to your spine as you engage your pelvic floor, drawing up through the centre of your body. Rise up on your toes, pushing your big toes firmly into the floor.

3 Inhale and hold the position. If you feel at all unsteady, stand next to a wall to do this exercise and hold onto the wall with one hand.

4 Exhale. Slowly lengthen your heels back down to the floor, keeping a long, tall spine.

reminders: Stand tall and, using all your toes, keep your weight evenly balanced on both feet.

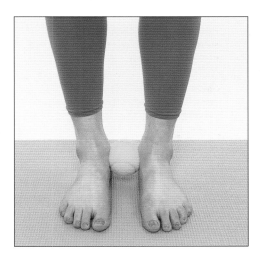

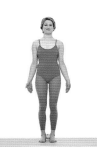
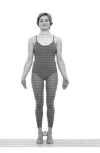
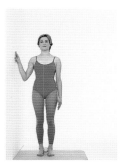
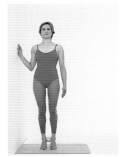

standing leg raise prep

aims

to learn balance; to find and hold correct alignment with each leg;
to strengthen the standing leg; and to learn how to stabilize the pelvis.

1 Stand in correct alignment, with your spine
long, your legs strong, your feet slightly apart
and your arms hanging straight down at each
side. Inhale and lengthen up through the spine.
Find a focus point ahead of you at eye level,
such as a window pane or a picture, as this
will help you to balance without wobbling.

2 Exhale and engage your pelvic floor by pulling
your navel in towards your spine as you bring
your right knee up towards your chest, holding
it with both hands. Keep your spine and standing
leg straight and strong and your hips level. You
will need to drop your right hip down and lift
the hip higher on the left side. Do not lean to
either side. Keep your torso square and your
shoulders level. Hold for a few breaths, and then
repeat with the other leg.

reminders: The body is upright so strong
abdominal control is needed. Stay centred.

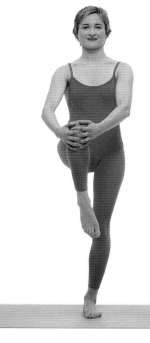

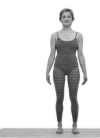
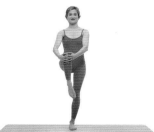

***chiropractor's
comments***
Great for working on balance,
lower body awareness and
control. Keep your pelvis
completely level and stable
at all times.

scapular awareness

aims

to help you become aware of how your shoulders work, and to isolate
the lower trapezius muscles used to stabilize the shoulder blades.

1 Stand facing a wall, about 15 cm (6 in) away, with
your feet parallel and hip-width apart. Your arms
should be bent so that your forearms and hands
are against the wall, just wider than shoulder-
width apart, palms facing each other, your thumbs
pointing away from the wall and your fingertips
at eye level. Inhale and lengthen the spine.

2 Exhale. Engage the navel to the spine and draw
your shoulder blades down towards the waist
as you slide your hands down the wall until your
fingertips are just below chin level. Inhale and

> **chiropractor's comments**
> The shoulder muscle's upper fibres are usually overtight, while
> the lower fibres tend to be weak, leading to 'winging' shoulder
> blades and bad posture – a source of upper back pain.

hold this position for a moment. Exhale. Then
slide your hands back to their starting position.
Repeat the sequence four times.

reminders: Don't lean into the wall as your
hands move downwards; stand tall, stay centred
and keep your neck long. Focus on the feeling
this exercise creates in your shoulder blades.

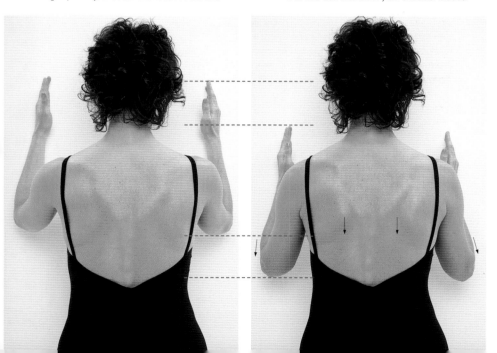

chicken wings with pole

aims

to learn correct use of the upper body; to open the chest and shoulders; to strengthen and stabilize the shoulders; and to maintain alignment within the body while moving the arms.

1 Stand in correct alignment, maintaining a long spine. Hold a pole with your hands just wider than shoulder-width apart and your arms relaxed. Inhale, and lengthen the spine. A broomstick makes a good pole for this exercise!

2 Exhale, draw your navel to your spine and stabilize as you raise the pole above your head, lifting your arms in front of you and keeping them straight – but with soft elbows. As you raise your arms, drop your shoulders down and away from your ears, and keep your elbows soft and your pelvis still.

3 Inhale. Then exhale and bend your arms to draw the pole down in front of you towards your chest. Feel your elbows and shoulder blades pull down to initiate the move. Keep the head in place and stand strong and tall.

chiropractor's comments
Keep your stomach muscles actively engaged and your sitting bones tucked under. Do not overarch your back. Feel the movement through your spine and shoulders.

4 Now inhale and slowly straighten the arms, raising the pole once again to its previous position over your head, as in step 2.

5 Exhale and bend your elbows to take the pole down behind your head. Feel your elbows and shoulder blades pull down to initiate the move. Keep your spine straight and your head and ribcage in place. Repeat the entire sequence four times.

reminders: Don't duck your head as you pull the pole downwards. Keep your body in alignment and make sure your arms move together rather than one arm being dominant.

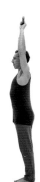
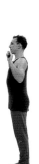
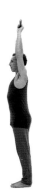

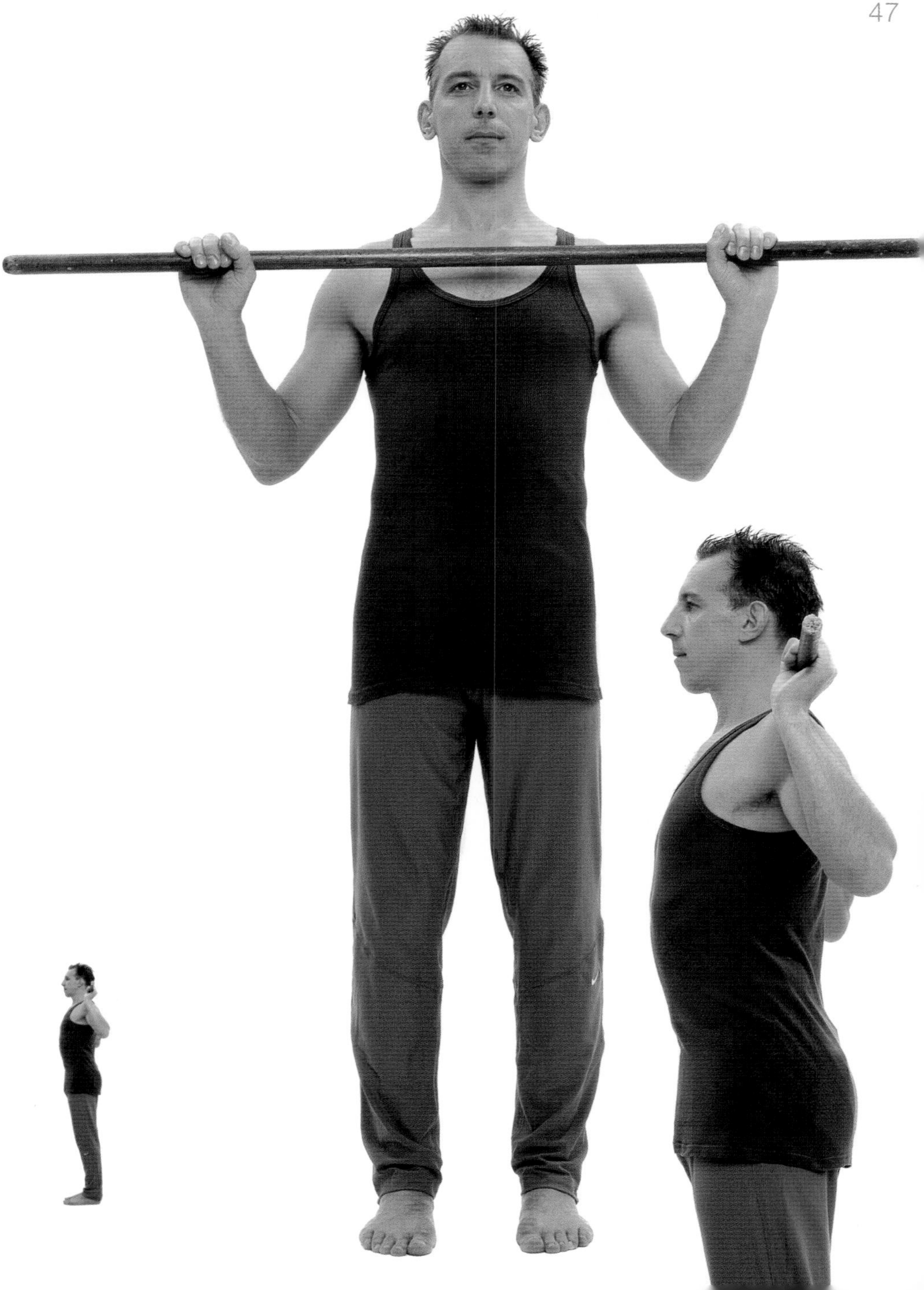

mountain pose to standing forward bend

aims

to build core strength and a strong foundation for correct standing alignment; to warm up the body and make contact with the body and the breath; to strengthen and lengthen legs; to open the upper body; and to stretch and strengthen the spine. Teaches the start of the sun salutation sequence.

1 Stand in correct standing alignment, samasthiti, as you did during the warm-up sequence (see samasthiti to mountain pose, page 26).

2 Inhale. Sweep your arms out and up from beside your thighs towards your head, palms facing down until your arms reach the halfway point.

3 Spin your palms up to face the sky as you finish the movement, bringing them together. Hold, if possible, with your hands above your head and gaze up at them, but keep your shoulders down. Lean backwards slightly, with the tailbone tucked under. Lift your arms high, lengthen the neck away from your chest and lengthen the front of the body.

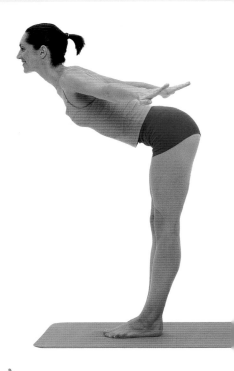

> **chiropractor's comments**
> Actively feel the relationship between the hamstrings and the motion of the lower back. Concentrate on the muscle balance of your erector spinae (lower back muscles) and your hamstrings. Please consult your doctor if you have a history of spinal or disc-related injury.

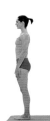
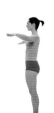
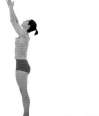
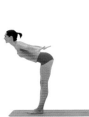

4 Exhale, sweep forward with a straight, lengthening spine, as if hinged at the hips. The arms sweep down, out and behind you like aeroplane wings.

5 Take your fingertips to the floor, or hold onto your ankles (as shown). Release your head from your shoulders so that it hangs down freely with the neck relaxed. Press your chest towards your thighs in a forward bend. Your hips should be directly above your heels. Straighten your legs if it is comfortable to do so without straining.

6 Inhale, sweep your arms out, back and up, to reverse the downward movement in step 4.

7 Return to the upward arms position in step 3. Repeat the entire sequence four times.

variations: If you feel your back beginning to round, bend your knees. People with tight hamstrings should use the bent-knee variation as they are more at risk of lower back injury in a forward bend. You can modify the stretch more by bending the knees as you bend forward, resting your elbows on your thighs. This allows you to lengthen the spine and feel stable without strain.

reminders: Press down evenly on both feet so that you are balanced. If you sway as you bend, move your feet further apart to stabilize yourself. Keep your hips directly over your thighs, knees, calves, ankles and feet to maintain body alignment. Hollow your stomach to lengthen the spine and keep your shoulders down, away from your ears.

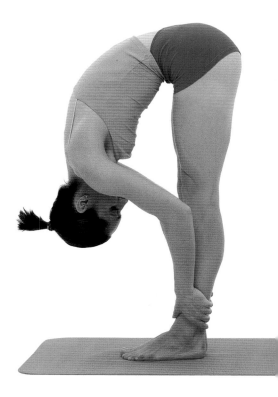

variations

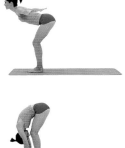

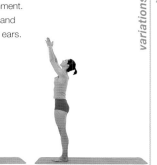

standing forward bend to lunge

aims

to build core strength and to improve circulation. The exercise involves strong abdominal work, which increases flexibility in the hips, spine and legs. Teaches another section of the sun salutation sequence.

1 Start by stretching and reaching into a forward bend position (see pages 48–9), with knees bent and palms to the floor.

2 Inhale and take your weight onto your left leg. Bend your right knee and bring it towards your face as the sole of your right foot points up and back to the ceiling.

3 Inhale and step back with your right leg into a lunge, keeping the right knee lifted off the floor and the leg as straight as possible. With the toes of the right foot on the floor, push back with the right heel and lift the back of the right thigh. There should be a right angle at your left knee, which should be directly above your left ankle, with your left thigh parallel to the floor. The tips of your fingers are placed slightly in front of the tips of your toes. The spine is straight and long.

Roll your shoulders back, away from your ears, and pull your shoulder blades down towards your waist. Look forwards and take a few breaths here.

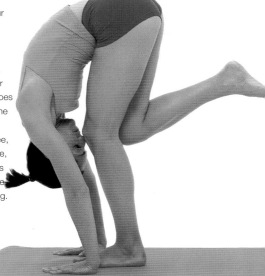

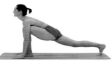

4 Exhale, then come forward into a forward bend as in step 2, stepping your right leg back under you to reverse the sequence.

5 Come back into the starting position, inhale and then repeat the forward bend into lunge with your left leg. Repeat four times, alternating legs.

reminders: Use your abdominals to lighten the weight on your fingertips. Keep your spine lifted and light. Don't allow your stomach to collapse onto your thigh.

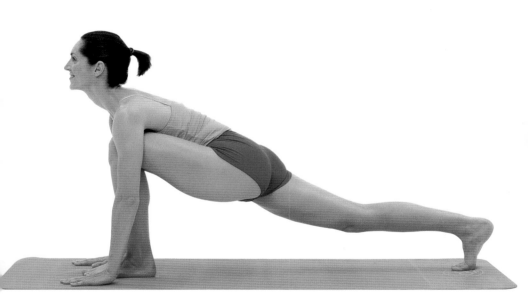

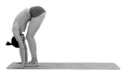

plank

aims

to build great strength in the biceps, triceps, shoulder and chest muscles and in the abdominals. As another part of the sun salutation sequence, this position teaches how to connect the strength of the entire body.

chiropractor's comments

This exercise builds strength for shoulder stabilization. But please use caution if you have a history of wrist injury, because it may put too much compressional force into your wrist joints. Stay strong and lifted through your abdominal muscles.

1 Start on your hands and knees. Don't arch your back but keep it straight and parallel to the floor instead, your spine long.

2 Inhale and extend your right leg out behind you, so that the leg is long and straight. Curl the toes under and rest them on the ground. Lift the back of the thigh and push your heel away from your hips. Find the connection from the buttocks down the back of the legs and out through the heel. The entire leg is engaged.

3 Keeping your hips stable, exhale and extend your left leg backwards, alongside your right leg. Maintain the strength in your legs. Lift the back of your thighs to the sky as you push out through both heels. Lift your stomach up to your spine, lift your kidneys upwards, and engage your inner thighs and your inner buttocks as you draw up through the centre of your body

to connect your legs, hips and stomach with your upper body work. Hold for 30 seconds, and then repeat three times.

reminders: Place your hands directly under the shoulders. Don't raise your hips too high or drop them down too low. Your hips should be lower than your shoulders but higher than your heels. Keep practising this one and you will succeed!

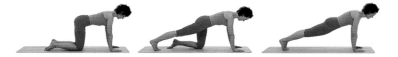

plank/dog/triangle

aims

to create a flowing sequence; to improve circulation; to build awareness of alignment; to develop strength and flexibility, building up the legs, hips and buttocks; and to open the chest and back.

1 Begin in plank pose (see steps 1–3 of plank, opposite). Keep your legs together and strong, your toes curled under and push out through your heels. Keep all muscles working together to connect through the upper and lower body and maintain a strong position.

chiropractor's comments

Great for opening and restoring movement and function to the spine. Keep the buttocks lifted and strong. Feel the head relax and drop away. Don't overload the shoulders and wrist joints. Please seek advice from your doctor if you have a history of wrist or shoulder problems.

2 Exhale and lift up into the dog pose. Lift your hips up to the sky, moving your shoulders away from your hands. Drop your heels down towards the floor. Straighten out your spine and arms and, if possible, your legs, too. You will have to maintain strength in your legs and stomach in order to make the transition smooth. Take a few breaths in this position to stabilize and prepare for step 3 (continued on page 54).

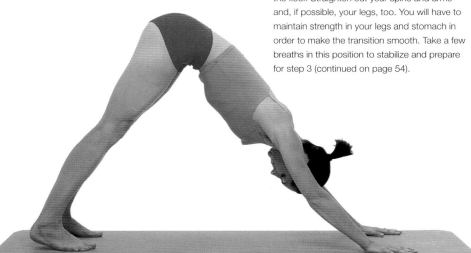

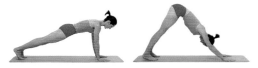

plank/dog/triangle

aims

to create fluidity; to develop strength and flexibility; to build alignment awareness; to improve circulation; to build the legs, hips and buttocks.

3 From dog pose, exhale and step forward with your left foot into a lunge, bringing your toes level with and just inside your left hand. Keep your chest open, the spine straight and your shoulders back, Your fingertips touch the floor on either side of the left foot. Take a few deep breaths to stabilize.

4 Inhale, straighten your left leg and push the heel of the back foot strongly into the floor, turning out the foot at an angle of about 45 degrees. Rest the left hand lightly on the left shin. Sweep your right hand up with a strong, long straight arm, the palm open and the fingertips reaching up.

The heel of your left foot should be in line with the arch of your right foot, and both feet should be pressed firmly into the floor. Lengthen the spine, sending the hips back, away from the shoulders, Keep the hips facing forwards, and scoop your tailbone down and under. Your inner thighs rotate outwards, away from each other. Keep your chest open and your

shoulders back – especially the right one – and your arms open wide from hand to hand. Reach right up with your right arm; be careful not to collapse onto the hand resting on your left shin. Look up at your right hand, if you comfortably can. Pull your shoulder blades down towards your waist. Hold the pose for five breaths and then reverse the sequence, returning to plank. Repeat on the other side.

reminders: This pose is difficult. Your upper hip will want to roll forward and down. Imagine the body is in one plane, pressed between two plates of glass, Work strongly and you will find that you progress. If you have tight hamstrings, rest your left hand on a higher surface – some books or a yoga brick – or place your hand higher up on your leg, or bend the front knee slightly.

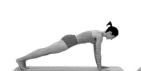

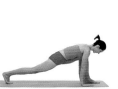
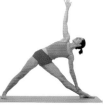

reverse tabletop

aims

to open the chest; to open and strengthen the shoulders; and to strengthen the back of the body.

chiropractor's comments

This is a great exercise for opening the front of the shoulders and the ribcage. But please be careful not to hyperextend your wrist joints and seek advice from your doctor if you have a history of wrist or shoulder problems.

1. Sit up straight with your legs together, straight out in front of you. Lift your breastbone and draw your shoulder blades downwards. Lengthen up through the top of the head to keep the spine long. Place your hands about 30 cm (12 in) behind your hips, shoulder-width apart, palms down and fingertips pointing to your hips. Inhale.

2. Exhale and lift your hips and chest up to the sky. Press the soles of your feet into the floor to stretch your legs and reach down into the floor with all ten toes. Your body should form a long straight-ish line, from toes to neck. Don't let your head drop backwards, which would compress the vertebrae. Instead, to lengthen the neck, tip the head slightly backwards and look forwards.

3. If step 2, which is the full pose – with lifted hips and straight legs – feels too difficult, simply modify it by bending your legs. From the sitting position, bend your knees, and move your feet back towards your buttocks until they are directly under the knees. Lift your hips and chest so that your spine is parallel to the floor, your shoulders are rolled back, your arms are straight and your hands are directly under your shoulders. Look forwards.

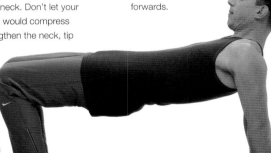

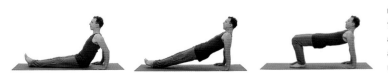

reminders: Keep your thighs strong, your armpit/chest area lifted and your shoulders rolled back.

backstroke

aims

to learn core stability, with a strong, stable torso holding still while the arms move; and to lengthen the spine.

1 Place a thin pillow under your head and lie in the relaxation pose, starting the neutral pelvis/ neutral spine alignment, with your arms at your sides, and the palms down on the floor. Inhale.

2 Exhale and engage, as you draw your navel back to the spine – and remembering to maintain alignment. Lift your right arm up to the sky and then continue back towards the floor behind you, without actually touching the floor. Keep alignment and keep the back of your ribcage down on the floor.

3 Inhale and bring your right arm back up to the centre, palms forward and fingertips reaching up to the ceiling. Bring your left arm up to the same point, so that both your arms are straight above your chest, shoulder-width apart, with your palms facing your feet.

4 Exhale. Then take your left arm backwards and your right arm forwards, as you maintain alignment. The arms should be soft but long: don't lock your elbows. Move your shoulder blades down towards your waist. Keep the front of your ribcage low to the ground. Reverse and repeat four times.

reminders: Keep your arms wide, ensuring that as they reach back they do not touch your ears.

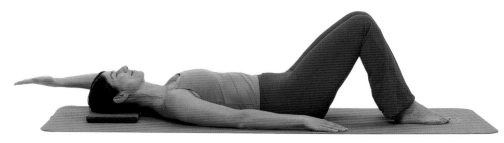

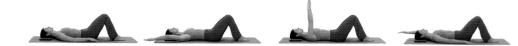

pelvic lifts

aims

to learn articulation of the spine, in order to increase flexibility and strength through the entire spine; to unlock areas of the spine, which may be very stiff; to increase space between each vertebra and to improve the health of the discs; and to strengthen the thighs and buttocks.

1 Lie in the relaxation pose, with your arms loosely down at your sides and your knees bent and your feet parallel, hip-width apart. Check your alignment. You can omit the pillow under your head, if desired. Inhale to prepare.

2 Exhale, engage the pelvic floor and draw your navel to the spine as you press your waist down to the floor. Lift your tailbone first, then your buttocks, your waist, your lower back, and then your middle back. Keep your shoulder blades firmly planted on the floor when you reach the highest point of the lift. You should be peeling one vertebra off the floor at a time as you roll up.

3 Inhale, hold the position, and prepare to roll back down. Exhale, reverse the movement and roll back down to your starting position, one vertebra at a time, dropping the ribcage down before your waist touches down and dropping the waist down before the hips touch down. Repeat the sequence four times.

chiropractor's comments
Activates gluteal muscles – one of the big culprits in lumbo-pelvic instability. A strong back needs strong buttocks. Concentrate on staying aware of your lower back and maintain a strong neutral pelvis and spine.

reminders: As you roll up off the floor, pull your knees away from the shoulders, lengthening the spine. As you roll back down to the floor, keep your hips as high as possible right up to the finish, as this stretches the spine well. Keep your weight pressed down and evenly distributed into both feet to minimize any slight swaying that may occur as you roll up or down. Set your hips down evenly. Don't lift too high when rolling up – your back should not arch and your ribcage should be relaxed at the highest point of the lift.

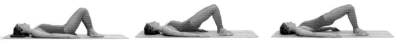

knee folds

aims

to learn how to keep the pelvis still and stable while the legs are lifted off the floor and moving; to develop concentration, focus and awareness; and to learn the importance of tiny movements!

chiropractor's comments
A small – but very important – exercise for the lower back. Keep the stomach muscles engaged and the lower back down.

1   Start in relaxation pose. Lie back in correct alignment with your arms at your sides, and a thin pillow beneath your head. Inhale to prepare.

2   Exhale and engage as you draw your navel in towards your spine. Lift your left heel, then slowly peel your whole foot off the floor, toes last, and, in a smooth movement, fold up your left knee until it is directly over your hip. Your toes should be pointing straight ahead, level with your knee, so that your shin is parallel to the floor. As you draw up your left knee, let the right thigh sink down into your right hip; keep your right hip down and your pelvis in neutral. You can place your hands on your hip bones to check that you are not tipping your pelvis when you move your legs. Press down equally on both buttocks into the floor.

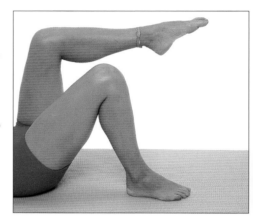

3   Exhale, and return to the starting position. Then work the other leg. Repeat four times on each leg, alternating legs.

reminders: There should be no wobbling in the pelvis as you lift or lower your leg. Slow down the movement if you do start to tremble. Keep your pelvis neutral throughout. Do not transfer your weight heavily onto the foot on the floor to stabilize but keep stable in your centre instead. Practise this one – it's more difficult than you think!

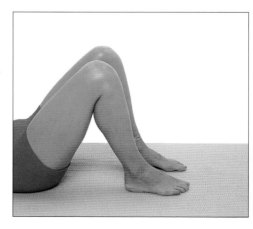

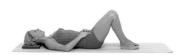

curl up

aims

to strengthen the deep abdominals and stretch the spine. A simple curl up can confirm whether or not you are engaging deep in the pelvic floor and deep abdominals. If you curl up keeping the pelvis neutral and see no bulge in your tummy, you are probably engaging correctly, which is good!

1 Lie in the relaxation position (no pillow needed for this exercise).

2 Interlock your fingers behind your head. Allow your elbows to come off the floor, pointing towards the sky but without squeezing your head. Inhale to prepare.

3 Exhale, engage as you draw your navel to your spine and curl your upper body forward. Take your chin towards your chest first, as you soften your breastbone down, and then peel the vertebrae off the floor one at a time. Keep your

chiropractor's comments

Watch the pressure that you put on your head and neck – you should really feel this exercise in your stomach, not your neck. Stomach muscles are very important for a strong lower back!

tailbone down, in contact with the floor, so that your pelvis stays in neutral. Look towards your pubic bone, and make sure that your stomach has not popped up! Inhale, reverse back down to your starting position and repeat four times.

reminders: Stay in neutral. Do not pull on your neck. Keep your chin a few inches off your chest. You should maintain a long, flat line from pubic bone to breastbone. Do not curl into a ball!

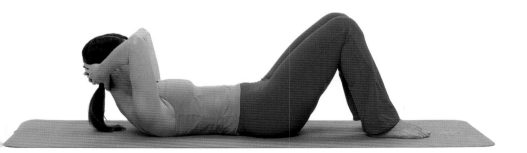

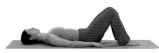
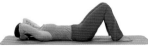
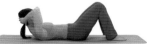

hundreds

aims

to learn breathing technique; to strengthen your deep abdominals; and to build core strength, keeping alignment strong, especially in shoulders. Increases circulation, and is often used as a warm-up in preparation for other exercises.

1 Start in the neutral pelvis/neutral spine position, with a thin pillow under your head, and your arms down at your sides. Begin to breathe deeply into your ribcage: inhale for a count of five, and exhale for a count of five and pump your arms up and down at your sides, lifting them about 15 cm (6 in) off the floor. Inhale deeply into the lower ribcage, expanding the ribcage for a count of five as you pump your arms to the count and then exhale fully for a count of five, still pumping your arms in time with your counting. Repeat.

2 Now, on an exhale, fold up one leg, bringing the knee up towards your chest until it is directly above your hip bone. Make sure you keep your pelvis still as you do so.

3 Fold up the other leg, so that both knees are directly above your hip bones, and your feet are at the same height as your knees, with the shins parallel to the floor. Point your toes and squeeze your inner thighs together. Keep your arm beats and the deep breathing pattern going.

4 Working on an exhale, curl your upper body forward, taking your chin towards your chest. Keep your shoulder blades down, and your pelvis in neutral, as you did in the previous exercise. Keep your shoulders away from your ears as you continue to pull down the shoulder blades towards your waist. Squeeze your inner buttocks and inner thighs to help stabilize yourself, continue to pull your navel back towards your spine and try to keep your lower legs parallel to the floor. Keep your arms beating up and down and keep the breathing pattern going until you have counted to 100, maintaining strong alignment throughout. Now fold one leg at a time back down to the floor. And finally release your head, neck and shoulders.

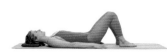
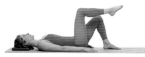
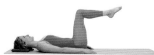

reminders: If you feel any strain on your neck, place one hand behind your head to support it, and then alternate arms until you've finished. Keep pulling your shoulder blades down towards your waist as your arms lengthen away from your shoulders. Focus on your pubic bone, and watch to see that your stomach does not bulge out. Keep your chest open, and a slight space between your chin and your chest so that you don't put any strain on your neck. Try to keep your breathing as relaxed as you can.

chiropractor's comments
This exercise is about stability and strength, so stay strong in your stomach and spine. Do not arch your lower back!

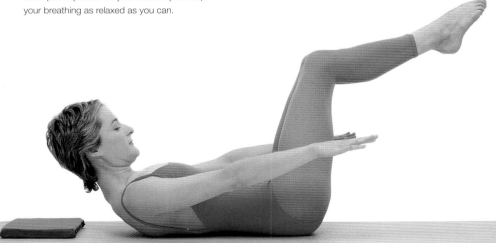

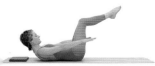

roll up with a band

aims

to build deep abdominal strength and stretch the spine; and to integrate the strength of the entire body – keeping it open, strong and long at the same time.

1 Start by sitting up tall, with your feet stretched away from you but your knees still bent, and yet your legs are long. Your feet are parallel and close together. Lift your pelvic floor and deep abdominal muscles so that you feel as if you can lift your buttocks off the floor. Keep that engagement, inhale and prepare to roll back.

2 Exhale, and keeping your navel drawn back to your spine, tip your pelvis backwards. Begin to roll back, pressing one vertebra at a time into the floor. As you roll back, keep your arms open and your elbows soft, and look forwards. Check to see that your stomach is not bulging upwards.

3 Roll back until your shoulders touch the floor, then release your neck, head and arms, letting them down onto the floor.

4 You are now correctly positioned to start coming back up. Inhale to prepare, exhale and reverse the movement, rolling back up

to a sitting position. First of all you bring your chin to your chest, then you lift your head, followed by the neck and shoulders. Keeping your arms long and open, and the elbows soft, complete the roll up by peeling one vertebra at a time off the floor – just check that your stomach is not sticking out!

reminders: While your feet should remain firmly planted on the floor throughout, your shoulder blades should be being continuously pulled down towards your waist. Release into the band as you roll up or down: as you engage your deep abdominals to keep the front of your body hollow, let your arms soften, so that the spine can relax and you can set down the vertebrae one by one. Keep the armpit/chest area open. Try not to touch your legs.

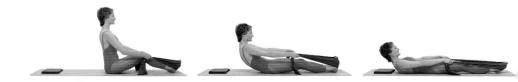

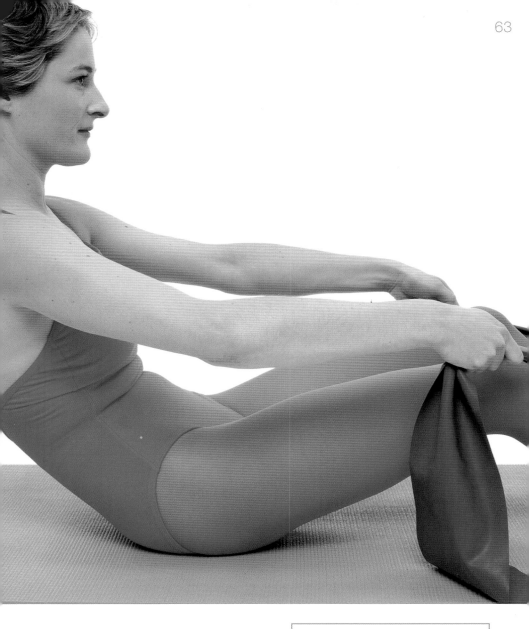

chiropractor's comments

Excellent for feeling the individual segmental motion of the
lumbar and thoracic spine. Roll down on a soft surface – a
mat, for example. Keep the neck long. Please consult your
doctor if you have a history of lower back injury.

swan dive prep

aims

to build control; to develop upper back strength; and to build deep abdominal strength to support the back in these moves. To integrate the strength of the entire body; to lengthen the spine; and to open the front of the body.

1 Begin by lying face-down on the mat, with your legs apart, keeping a long, neutral pelvis/neutral spine. Your elbows are bent, your forearms flat on the floor next to your ribcage, and your palms flat on the floor directly in front of your elbows. Your abdominals are strongly engaged, drawing your navel back to the spine; your stomach should not push into the floor. Hold the pubic bone down, tighten your buttocks and thighs, and engage your legs, your toes drawing away from your hips to lengthen your legs. Inhale to prepare.

2 Exhale, press down on your elbows and palms and lift your head, and then your shoulders and chest. Keep the elbows down on the floor at first and your shoulder blades drawn back and down.

chiropractor's comments

Excellent for building strength and flexibility in the back extensor muscles – and great for strengthening the buttocks! Don't overarch if there is any feeling of discomfort. Please consult your doctor if you have, or have had, a disc- or spine-related problem.

3 As you lift yourself higher your elbows will come off the floor and your arms will straighten, but keep your shoulders down and away from your ears. Lift your chest high. Your legs need to work hard in support: point your toes, and pull your legs away from your hips.

4 Inhale, and reverse the movements to come back down to your starting position. Repeat the sequence four times.

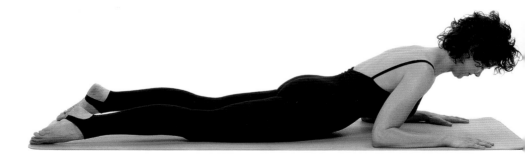

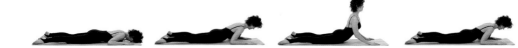

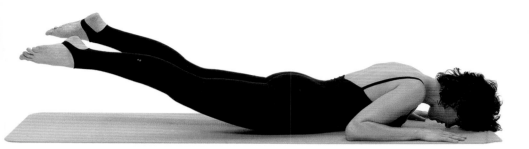

5   Exhale. Press down into your elbows and palms, fingers spread, in order to stabilize your upper back and shoulders before you lift your legs off the floor. Keep your stomach hollow and lifted towards your spine.

6   Lift your legs off the floor, but continue to press down on the elbows and palms, stabilizing the shoulders, and pulling the shoulder blades down towards your waist. Your forehead should remain resting on the floor, so that you are looking down at the floor, and your neck should stay long.

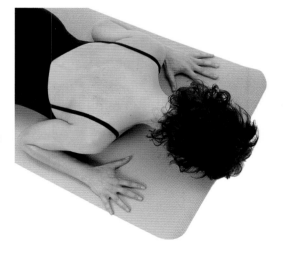

7   Continue to lift your legs away until your thighs are off the ground – but only if you feel no discomfort. Hold and inhale, then reverse the sequence to return to your starting position. Repeat four times.

reminders: Keep your stomach lifted throughout the sequence, and your buttocks and the back of your legs strongly engaged. You should not feel any pain in your lower back.

  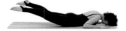

side leg lifts

aims

to work from a strong centre, which remains stable as you raise and lower the legs; to improve balance; and to tone hips, buttocks, thighs and stomach.

chiropractor's comments
Great for working medial and lateral thighs and gluteal muscles – common culprits in lower back and pelvic pain syndromes.

1
Lie on your right side in alignment, your spine on the back edge of the mat, your feet out at the front edge. Place your left palm flat on the floor in front of your ribcage while your right arm supports your head. Keep both your shoulders back and your chest open. Your left hip should be directly over your right hip, your left shoulder directly above your right shoulder, and your top leg on the lower leg, with both your toes softly pointed. Inhale to prepare.

2
Exhale. Pull your navel to your spine as you engage your pelvic floor and lift both legs off the floor. Press one leg against the other so both remain active. Only lift your legs to just above hip height, then lower them to just below hip height. Keep your waist off the floor at all times. To learn control, draw your legs away from the hips trying to extend their length rather than increasing the height of your lift. Inhale, lower your legs and repeat ten times.

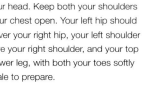

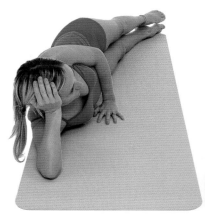

reminders: Slow controlled lifts and lowers of the legs. Pull your navel to your spine, keep your chin away from your chest, and keep your chest open and your shoulders back.

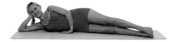

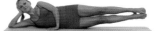

dead bug

aims

to stretch the hips, hamstrings, inner thighs and lower back.

1 Lie on your back and bring your knees to your
chest. With your thumbs facing your heels, take
hold of the inner edge of your feet. The soles of
your feet should face the ceiling. Lift your heels
and pull your toes down. Gently pull your knees
down towards your armpits, but keep your hips
down on the floor. Lengthen your spine.

reminders: Breathe comfortably. Keep your
neck long and on the floor, and your head on
the floor. Your ankles should stay directly
above your knees, and your spine
should drop into closer and closer
contact with the floor.

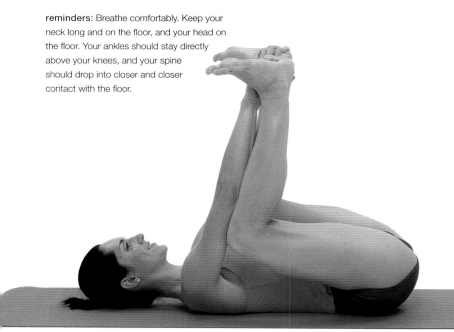

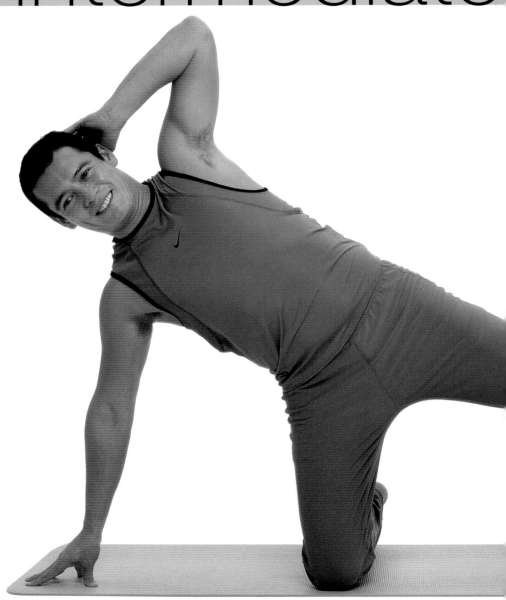

intermediate

programme

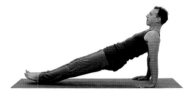

The intermediate programme assumes that you can engage the pelvic floor, perform lateral breathing, find correct alignment, and that you can easily complete the beginner's programme in a relaxed manner – and are able to work from a strong centre with good control. These exercises challenge your strength a bit more; they become more complex and demand more precision. Take your time and work on fine-tuning. Before you begin, complete the three warm-ups (see pages 34–7) and carefully read the instructions and look at the sequences for each exercise.

freestanding roll down

aims

to relax the spine, increasing the space between each vertebra and allowing the discs to expand and the spine to lengthen; to relax the shoulders and chest to create flexibility and strength in the spine; to learn spinal articulation; to strengthen abdominals and build core strength.

> **chiropractor's comments**
> This exercise involves forward flexion and stability of the lower back; see your doctor if you have any disc-related problems. As you bend forward, feel each segment of your spine stretching apart, one by one, removing any stiffness.

1 Stand in alignment with your feet parallel and hip-width apart. Keep your knees relaxed. Inhale and lengthen your spine.

2 Exhale, release your head and neck, and begin to roll forward, softly dropping your chin towards your chest. Let the weight of your head carry you down, rolling through your spine like a wheel, one vertebra at a time. Keep your hips in place and let your arms dangle like a puppet, without tension.

3 As you roll down to the floor, lift your navel higher towards your spine so that the front of your body feels lifted, helping to open the back of your body. Inhale. Exhale and reverse to come back up to standing, rolling one vertebra at a time and dropping down your tailbone. Your head, neck and shoulders should be the last to come up.

reminders: Try to roll down through the centre of your body and avoid swaying from side to side. Make sure that your weight is evenly balanced.

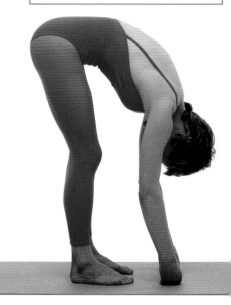

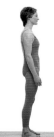
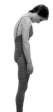

standing pelvic tilts

aims

to increase flexibility and strength in the spine; to build strength in the lower abdominals; to wake up the lower back area.

1 Stand with your feet parallel and hip-width apart. Bend your knees as you lean forwards, with your hands resting on your thighs. Keep your spine long and flat, and drop your shoulders away from your ears. Inhale, lengthen the spine and send your sitting bones/buttocks up towards the sky. Roll your shoulders back and look up as you form a c-curve with your spine. Your legs should remain in the same fixed position throughout.

2 Exhale and reverse the above movement, creating a c-curve in the opposite direction as your chin tucks down towards your chest. Contract your abdominal muscles and lift, navel to spine, so that your pubic bone tucks forward towards your chest. Keep your legs still throughout.

reminders: As your pelvis tilts back and forth, the entire spine is involved in the movement. Try to avoid changing the position of your legs.

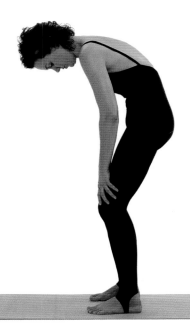

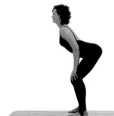
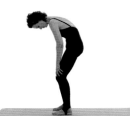

chiropractor's comments

Gently flex and extend your middle and lower spine. Stay within a pain-free range of movement to warm up the back gently. Feel the spine come alive, becoming more supple and active!

standing leg raise

aims

to learn balance; to find and hold correct alignment with each leg; to strengthen the standing leg; to stabilize the pelvis; to stretch the back of the legs; and to build hip flexors.

1 Stand in correct alignment, with your spine long, legs strong, feet slightly apart and arms straight down at your sides. Inhale and lengthen up through your spine. Find a focus point ahead of you at eye level, as staring at this will help you keep your balance. Move your left hand to your left hip.

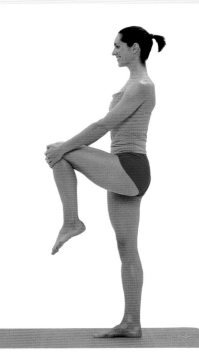

2 Exhale and engage the pelvic floor by pulling your navel in towards your spine as you bring the left knee up towards your chest. Hold the knee with both hands, keeping your spine straight and your standing leg straight and strong.

Keep your hips level – you will have to drop your hip down on the raised leg side and lift your hip higher on the standing leg side. Stay centred – do not lean to either side. Keep your torso square and your shoulders level.

3 Exhale, and extend your left leg straight out in front of you at hip height, holding onto the back of your thigh to support it.

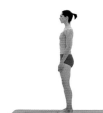
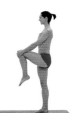
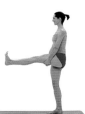
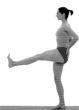

4 Now release your arms, and rest them on your buttocks, but keep the leg extended in front of you, at hip height. Keep your standing leg straight and strong, your hips level and your spine long. Lift your chest. Hold for 20 seconds, and then slowly lower your leg to the floor. Repeat to raise your right leg.

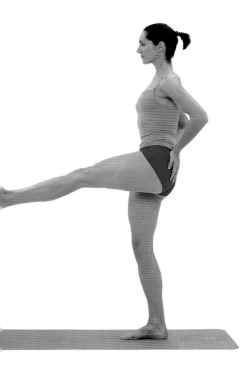

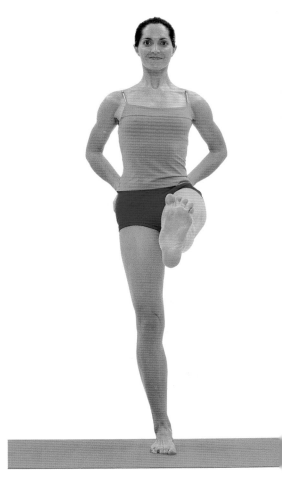

reminders: The body must be upright throughout the exercise, and strong abdominal control is needed to stay centred.

chiropractor's comments

Keep your pelvis level, preventing one side from rising up. Feel the lower back muscles, like two ropes on each side of the spine, stabilizing and controlling. This is great for toning and strengthening the anterior thighs and hip flexors.

Before performing this exercise complete
mountain pose to forward bend on pages 48–9.

child's pose to dog

aims

to lengthen the spine, strengthen the arms and open the shoulders; to tone the legs, work the feet and relax the mind. This is true power yoga, working on breathing and overall flexible strength in a flowing sequence: a rest pose, a transition and then a strong pose – the dog pose.

1 Kneel with the tops of your feet flat on the floor and your knees wide apart. Shift your hips back so that your buttocks are in contact with your heels. Stretch your arms out in front of you and walk your hands forwards, dropping your ribcage down to the floor, lengthening your spine and taking your forehead down last, to touch the floor.

You may find that you cannot sit down on your heels, but try to maintain a hip–heel contact with your spine long and straight. There should be no pressure on your neck and head; your weight should fall back onto your heels.

chiropractor's comments

Feel the shoulders release; be careful of hyperextending them. Slowly warm up the stretch. Feel the spine lengthen and be aware of the head and pelvis pulling away from each other.

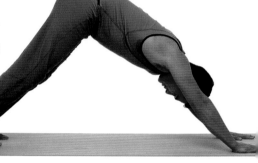

2 Inhale. Maintain the distance between your hands and feet as you slowly come up onto your hands and knees, adjusting your feet to be hip-width apart.

3 Exhale, curl your toes under, lift your hips to the sky and straighten your legs, moving into the dog pose (see also page 77). Straighten your spine, legs and arms, and pull the shoulders away from your hands – shoulder blades placed firmly down on the back of your ribcage. Lift your sitting bones, pull your hips and thighs further backwards to lengthen the waist, and fully extend your arms, dropping your heels to the floor if possible.

4 Inhale and come down again onto your hands and knees. Exhale, returning to your starting position – known as the child's pose – and repeat the whole sequence four times.

reminders: If your hamstrings are tight, your spine will not be straight and this will put strain on the discs. By bending your legs in the dog pose you can fully lengthen the spine and release your lower back. In the dog pose, try bending and then straightening your legs to observe the relationship between the spine, pelvis and legs.

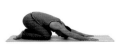
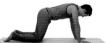
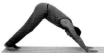
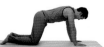

forward bend to plank

aims

to build flexible strength; to learn the 'flight pattern' – the lightness of lifting your hips high and your feet off the floor; to build core strength, stabilize the shoulders and build upper- and lower-body integration; and to strengthen the arms.

1 Starting in correct alignment, proceed smoothly into a forward bend (see steps 4 and 5 of mountain pose to forward bend on page 49).

2 Now bend your knees and exhale to draw the navel back to the spine. Lift the hips high and shoot your legs out behind into plank. The jump is light and easy, so be sure to land lightly: float backwards, as if in slow motion. Only with much practice will this weightless quality be achieved!

3 In the plank pose your hands are directly under your shoulders, palms flat on the floor, fingers evenly spread, and hands shoulder-width apart.

> **chiropractor's comments**
> Consult your doctor if you have any wrist-, shoulder- or disc-related problems. Keep a firm stance through your hands and shoulder joints, and then proceed to jump. Practise slowly to prevent any injury. This is great for balance and coordination!

Maintain the strength in your legs. Lift the backs of your thighs to the sky as you push out through both heels. Now lift your stomach towards the spine, lift your lower back up, and engage your inner thighs and buttocks as you draw up through the centre of your body to connect the work of your legs, hips and stomach with your upper-body work. Look down at your hands, keeping your neck long. Breathe, hold for 30 seconds and then repeat the exercise three times.

reminders: This exercise works all the muscles, so it's worth practising and getting it right! Keep your hands directly under your shoulders and your hips stable and straight, lower than your shoulders but higher than your heels.

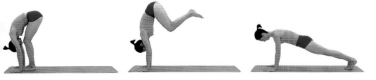

plank with knee to chest

aims

to build deep core and upper-body strength, and strong abdominals; to find the connection of integrated body strength, learning to work every muscle in the body. This is a flowing sequence of connected poses that builds deeper strength.

1 Start by assuming the dog pose (see steps 1–3 of child's pose to dog on page 74). Hold for several deep breaths.

2 Exhale, and extend your right leg up and out to the sky behind you. Take a few deep breaths in the pose.

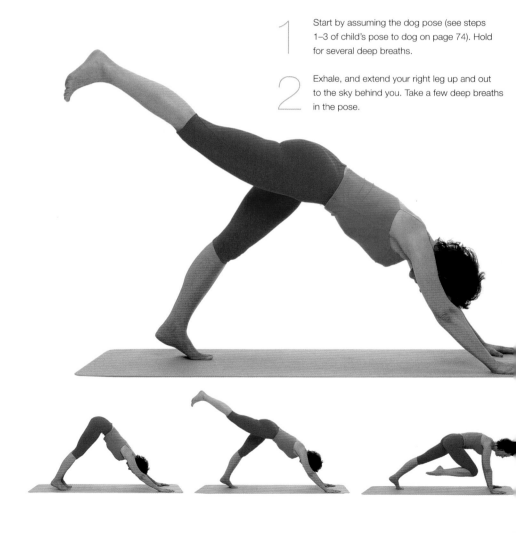

3 Exhale and, holding strong in your centre and in your shoulders, bring your right knee forwards to your chest, lifting your hips and spine upwards and sending your shoulders forwards so that they are directly over your hands. Keep your stomach hollow to build strength and to accommodate the rising knee. Keep your right foot lifted high off the floor with your toes pointed to the wall behind you.

Pushing strongly into the ball of your foot, lift your back heel off the floor, and extend your heel so that your supporting leg is strong and you feel a connection from your heel to the back of your leg and buttocks, through to your spine and abdominals, to your shoulders. Take five deep breaths in this pose.

4 In order to return to the dog pose, and from there to reverse the whole sequence, exhale and extend your right leg out behind you again.

5 Lower your right leg and adopt the dog pose, your starting position. Repeat the sequence three times, working each leg alternately.

reminders: The dog pose is a fabulous yoga posture. You will probably spend the rest of your life enjoying it and working on improving it. Experiment with it to discover your strong arms, long spine, long legs and high hips. Breathe deeply during this sequence, because the exercise is challenging and requires strength and focus. The entire body is at work here. If you want to work the spine a little harder, try bending and straightening your legs in the stretch.

chiropractor's comments
This is a great sequence for coordinating strength, endurance and flexibility through the hips and lumbo-pelvic regions. Keep stable and level in the pelvis.

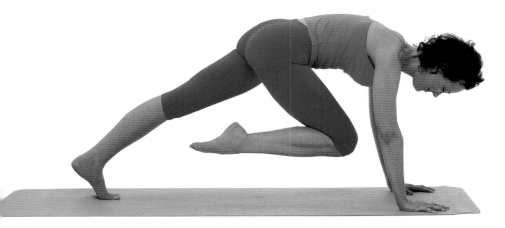

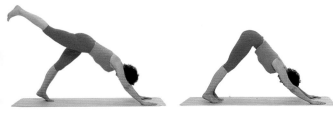

dog into warrior 1

aims

to increase strength in the legs and find flexibility in the hips; to improve core strength; to lengthen the spine; to open the chest and shoulders; and to stretch the arms, hands and wrists. The connected sequence of poses will build a fluid strength and flexibility.

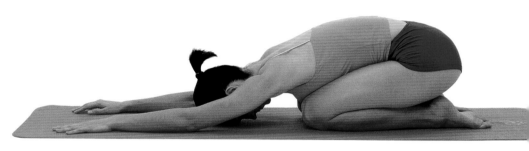

1 Start in the child's pose (see step 1 of child's pose to dog on page 74), with palms, forehead, knees and tops of feet to the floor.

2 Inhale and move forwards onto your hands and knees. Be careful not to arch your back, which should be parallel with the floor.

3 Exhale and lift your body slowly up into the dog pose (see step 3 on page 74). Curl your toes under and lift your hips to the sky, feet shoulder-width apart, heels to the floor. Straighten your spine, legs and arms, and pull your shoulders away from your hands, shoulder blades firmly down on the back of your ribcage. Lift up your sitting bones, lengthen the waist by pulling back your hips and thighs, and fully extend your arms.

4 From the dog pose, exhale and lunge your left foot forwards, placing it between your hands, making an angle of 90 degrees (a right angle) at your front knee. Turn out your back foot by about 45 degrees. Your front heel should be in line with the instep of your back foot.

5 Inhale and, taking your hands off the floor and straightening up so that your weight is more evenly distributed between your front and back legs, sweep your arms out to the sides and up to shoulder height. Turn your right foot outwards and lower your heel to the floor. Keep centred and strong with your arms directly out to the sides and parallel with the floor. Lengthen your spine, lift your chest and draw your ribcage back above your hips in a straight line.

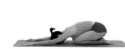
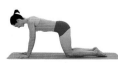
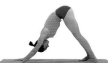
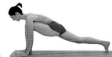

6 Now raise your arms to the sky in a sweeping movement so that your arms finish up at each side of the head. The arms are straight, parallel to each other, with palms facing. Keep your arms close to your ears. Drop your shoulder blades down, away from your ears. Keep your chest lifted and your ribcage drawn back above your hips in a straight line. Pull down your tailbone, and lift the top of your head. The spine is long. Lift your stomach up and away from the front thigh. Make sure your hips are square to the front, rotating to pull your left hip back and the right hip forward.

Drop your hips down: your front thigh should be parallel to the floor (see close-up, above right). Press down into your back heel, and the outer edge of your back foot, lifting your inner ankle, and keep your back leg active and strong. Look straight ahead. Reverse back through the sequence to return to the dog pose, and repeat on the other side.

reminders: Your shin and the thigh of your front leg should form a right angle. Lift right up to the sky with the spine and arms!

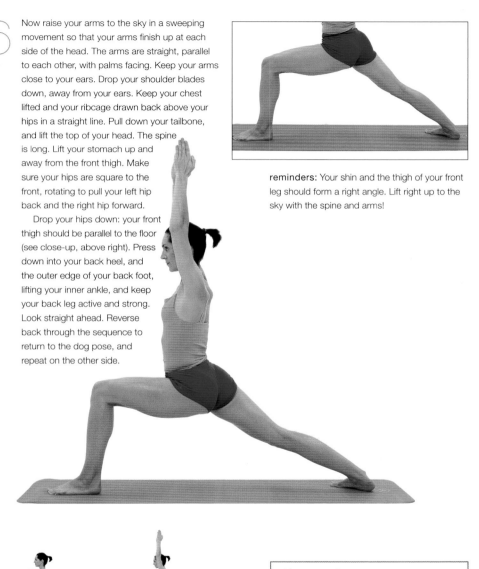

chiropractor's comments

This sequence opens the pelvis and restores movement through the hip, but be careful with your knees. Be aware of the position of your back leg, and do not put excessive medial strain/rotation on the knee joint.

warrior 1 into warrior 2

aims

to build core strength; to open hips; and to strengthen and tone buttocks, thighs, shoulders, arms, abdominals and deep spinal muscles. This is another connected sequence which gives a taste of the flowing movement of a sequence of postures.

> **chiropractor's comments**
> This pose opens the pelvis and stretches the anterior hip flexors. Feel the deep spinal muscles lifting and engaging.

1   Warrior 2 develops from warrior 1 so, first of all, follow steps 1–6 on pages 78–9, to work from the dog pose to warrior 1.

2   Now turn your hips and shoulders to face the side, leaving your feet in position. The front leg is still at a right angle with your knee directly over your heel, with your thigh parallel to the floor.

3   Drop your arms down to shoulder level until they are parallel to the floor, with palms down. Your front arm should be over your front thigh, your back arm in line with your back leg. Reach through the middle fingers, as if the arms are being pulled in opposite directions. Look at your front hand. The stretch fingertip to fingertip is long. Now return to warrior 1 and dog (see pages 78–9) before repeating on the other side.

reminders: Keep both feet firmly planted on the mat. Lift your stomach, spine and chest, but keep your shoulders down and your front thigh low.

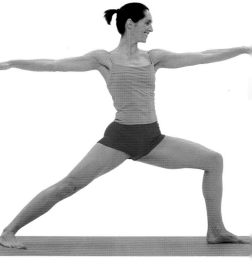

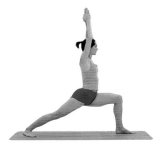

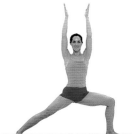

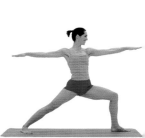

reverse plank

aims

to build core strength; to open the chest and open and strengthen the shoulders; to strengthen the back of the body; and to stretch the legs.

1 Sit up straight with both your legs together straight out in front of you. Lift your breastbone and draw your shoulder blades down. Lengthen up through the top of your head to lift your spine. Place your hands about 30 cm (12 in) behind your hips, shoulder-width apart, palms down and fingertips pointing towards your hips. Inhale.

chiropractor's comments

Please see your doctor if you have any shoulder-related injuries. Protect your wrist and shoulder joints by making sure you do not hyperextend them too far. This is a great exercise for strengthening your gluteal muscles, shoulders and core stabilizers.

2 Exhale. Lift up your hips and chest towards the sky and stretch your legs, pressing down into your feet and reaching to the floor with all of your toes. Your body should be in a long straight line from toes through to neck. Try to lengthen the neck out of the chest by tipping your head slightly backwards to look straight ahead. Avoid dropping your head back, which compresses the vertebrae.

reminders: Hold your thighs strong, keep your shoulders rolled back and keep your armpit and chest lifted. If possible, keep your feet together and pull your toes to the floor.

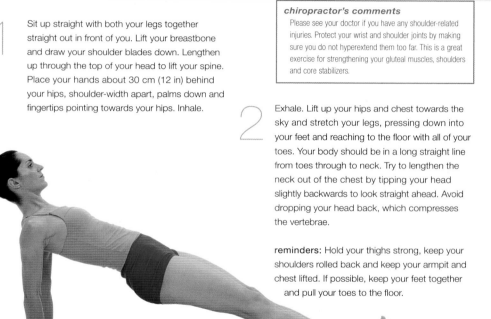

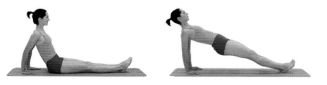

legs walk up the wall

aims

to develop integrated core strength, and a sense of lightness in the body when the feet leave the floor; to familiarize yourself with inversion postures; and to build upper body strength – all preparations for full handstands.

1 Sit up straight with your legs stretched out in front of you and your feet touching a wall. Mark the position of your hip bones by placing an object, such as a yoga brick, on the floor.

2 Leaving the marker in place, turn over onto your hands and knees. Place your hands level with the marker, with your palms flat down and place the soles of your feet against the wall.

3 Lift your left knee forward and your hips up so that you assume the pose of a runner on a starting block: knees off the floor, with your left knee close to your chest and the ball of the back foot against the wall.

4 Extend the right leg as high up the wall as possible. Maintain strong, straight arms and use your abdominal strength to keep your hips high.

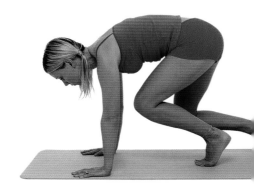

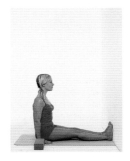
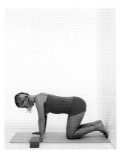
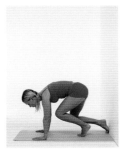
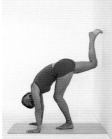

5 Extend your left leg up the wall. Stabilize by straightening your arms and lifting your shoulders away from your ears. Engage your pelvic floor, inner thighs and buttocks to lift your hips. Breathe and relax.

6 Now, keeping your arms strong, your shoulders lifted and your hips light and lifted, walk your feet down the wall until the thighs are parallel to the floor, making your body into an angle of 90 degrees. Stabilize the pose, relax and breathe deeply! Hold for 20 seconds.

reminders: Keep your spine long, your arms straight, your shoulders away from your ears and your hips lifted high.

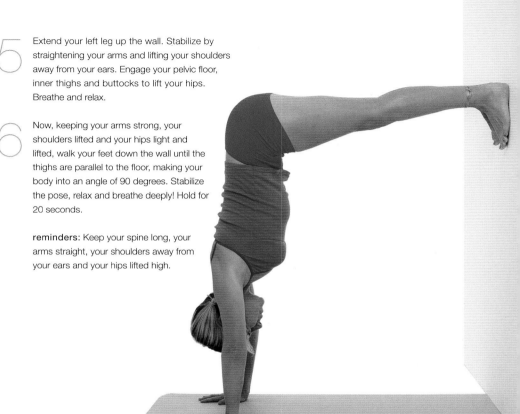

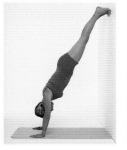

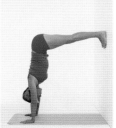

chiropractor's comments

While this is a good exercise for working the upper back and shoulders, please consult your doctor if you have a history of disc or shoulder injuries. Maintaining control prevents injury, so stay lifted and tight in the abdominal muscles to prevent any twisting of the spine or hips.

arm openings

aims

to open and stabilize the upper body; to stretch the chest, the sides of the body and the arms; and to create a gentle rotation in the spine. The exercise will also improve your breathing technique.

1 Lie on your side with a thin pillow beneath your head. Bring your knees up to make an angle of 90 degrees at your hip, with your feet directly under your knees, your lower leg forming an angle of 90 degrees with your thighs. Your spine is straight, keeping its natural curves, with your shoulders aligned directly above the hip bones. Reach your arms out in front of you at shoulder level, with palms together. Keep the neck long and the chin away from the chest. Inhale to prepare.

2 Breathe out and engage the pelvic floor. Inhale and reach up with the top arm, lifting the fingertips to the ceiling and turning to look at your raised hand. Keep your shoulder blades down.

3 Exhale and, with the same arm, reach back to the floor behind you, turning your head to watch your hand. Aim to reach the floor, but only if you can do so easily, keeping your knees together, your hips in their starting position and your stomach hollow.

chiropractor's comments
A gentle opening of the ribcage and thoracic spine – great for releasing tightness in the upper back. Feel the movement between the shoulder blades and the spine. This exercise also involves rotation of the lower spine, so please seek advice from your doctor if you feel any discomfort.

reminders: Keep your ribcage low to the floor as you take your arm behind you. Lengthen the waist and spine. Concentrate on working your deep abdominals throughout.

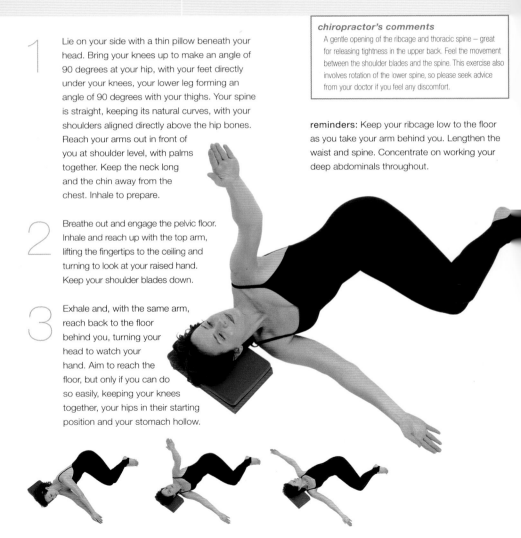

pelvic lifts squeezing a yoga block

aims

to increase flexibility and strength through the entire spine, and to gently unlock areas of the spine which may be stiff by moving the spine vertebra by vertebra; to improve the health of the discs; to strengthen the thighs and buttocks; and to work the inner thighs.

chiropractor's comments

As you activate and lift your pelvis, keep your neck and upper back relaxed. This is a great pose for opening and strengthening the lower spine and buttocks.

1 Lie in the relaxation pose with your arms loosely by your sides and your feet parallel, hip-width apart. Check alignment. Place a pillow or yoga block between your knees. Inhale to prepare.

2 Exhale. Then engage your pelvic floor, draw your navel to your spine and squeeze the pillow between your knees. Press your waist to the floor and then, in order, lift your tailbone, buttocks, waist, lower back, and finally your middle back, peeling one vertebra off the floor at a time, and coming up to your highest point with your shoulder blades still firmly planted on the floor.

Inhale, hold the position and prepare to roll down again. Exhale and roll back down to your starting position, dropping one vertebra at a time, making sure that you drop the ribcage down before the waist touches the floor and you drop the waist before the hips touch. Repeat the sequence four times.

reminders: Squeeze the pillow throughout the exercise. As you roll up, pull your knees away from your shoulders. As you roll down, keep your hips as high as possible until the finish. Press down into your feet and keep your weight evenly distributed: this will help to correct any slight sway. Avoid arching your back; your ribcage should be relaxed at the highest point of the lift. Set your hips down evenly.

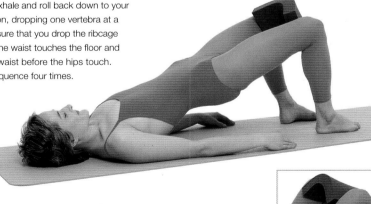

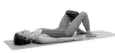
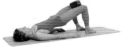

oblique curl up

aims

to strengthen the oblique abdominals and stretch the spine.

1 Lie in the relaxation position (see step 1 on page 85, but without a pillow or yoga block). Interlock your fingers behind your head and bring your elbows off the floor, so that they point to the sky, but do not squeeze your head. Inhale to prepare.

2 Exhale and engage as you draw your navel to your spine. Tip your head forwards, taking your chin towards your chest as you soften your breastbone down. Roll up slowly, peeling one vertebra at a time off the floor. Keep your tailbone in contact with the floor so that the pelvis stays in neutral position. Look towards your pubic bone, and check that your stomach has not popped up!

chiropractor's comments
Be careful of excessive pulling on your neck – you should feel the exercise targeting your stomach muscles.

3 Inhale, and rotate your trunk to the right from the waist, bringing your left armpit towards your right knee.

4 Exhale and extend your right arm, reaching away from your body as you pulse forward. Lean slightly back on inhale. Repeat five times. Imagine, as you pulse forward, reaching towards your extended arm, that there is a hinge at the 'bra line' from which you fold forward, lifting your right shoulder blade off the floor as you do so. Work each side four times.

reminders: Avoid rolling onto your right shoulder. Keep your tailbone down and stay in neutral position. Do not pull on your neck and keep your chin a few inches off your chest.

For a full extension of this exercise,
see **hundreds** on pages 60–1.

87

hundreds

aims

to learn good breathing technique; to warm up in preparation for other exercises, and improve circulation generally; to strengthen the deep abdominals; to keep strong alignment, especially in shoulders; and to stretch the legs.

1 Begin by following steps 1–3 of the full hundreds sequence on pages 60–1.

> ***chiropractor's comments***
> Strong abdominal musculature leads to a strong lower back, the primary support of the lumbar spine. To work the correct muscles, keep your lower spine flat.

2 On an exhale, curl your upper body forward taking your chin towards your chest, but keeping your shoulder blades down, your shoulders away from your ears, and the pelvis in neutral (as in the oblique curl up exercise, opposite). Engage your inner buttocks and inner thighs to stabilize as you press your navel back towards the spine. Your breathing and arm beats should continue.

3 On an exhale, straighten your legs, pointing your toes to the sky. Keep your arms beating and keep the regular breathing pattern going until you count to 100! Maintain strong alignment.

reminders: If you feel any strain in your neck, place one hand behind your head to support it, and then alternate arms until you have finished. Look at your pubic bone to check that your stomach is not bulging. Keep your chest open and a slight space between your chin and chest. Your breathing should be relaxed.

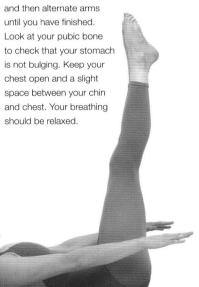

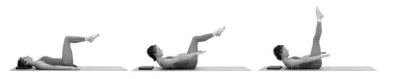

roll up

aims

to build deep abdominal strength; to give the spine a good stretch; and to integrate the strength of the entire body, keeping the body open, strong and long at the same time.

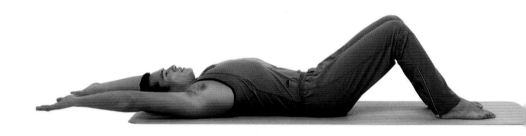

1 Lie down in the neutral pelvis/neutral spine relaxation pose, with your arms over your head and hovering just above the floor.

2 Inhale and slowly bring your arms up until they are directly above your shoulders, and perfectly straight.

3 On exhale move your arms forwards and simultaneously begin rolling your upper body forwards in one smooth motion, taking your chin to your chest first of all, then following by lifting your head, neck and shoulders off the floor. As you roll up your arms will come to rest below your knees in a straight line from the shoulders and parallel to the floor.

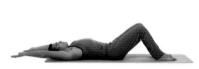
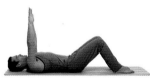
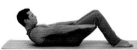

4 Now continue rolling up to lift your upper back and then your lower back, peeling one vertebra at a time off the floor. Keep your arms long and parallel to the floor, and your elbows soft, reaching away from the shoulders. Keep focusing on your stomach to check that it is not bulging out.

5 When you have fully rolled up, sit up tall, with your feet stretched away from you, slightly apart but parallel. Lift your pelvic floor, and engage the deep abdominal muscles so that you feel as if you can lift your buttocks off the floor. Keep the engagement and inhale. Prepare to roll back on an exhale. Reverse the movement so that you roll back down very slowly and with focus. Repeat four times.

reminders: Your feet should remain firmly planted on the floor throughout the roll up, and your shoulder blades should pull down continuously towards your waist. Let your arms become softer and engage your abdominals to keep the front of your body hollow – so that the spine can relax – and set down one vertebra at a time. Keep the armpit-chest area open.

chiropractor's comments
The exercise works both superficial and deep abdominal muscles – the strength centre of the body. Roll up gently through the lower back into the mid back.

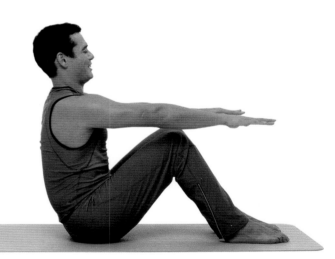

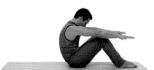
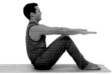

single leg stretch

aims

to build a strong stable centre which does not move when arms and
legs are moving; to improve coordination; to strengthen the deep
abdominals and buttocks; to lengthen the spine; and to improve your
breathing technique. This is an exercise of flowing movement.

1 Lie in the relaxation position with your knees
softly bent and your arms loosely by your sides.
Inhale to prepare.

2 Exhale, and engage the pelvic floor, drawing
your navel back to your spine. Then fold one
knee up towards your chest, until it is directly
above your hip bone, and your thigh is at an
angle of 90 degrees to the ground.

3 Now fold up the other knee so that both knees
are above your hip bones and your shins are
parallel to the floor – toes are touching, at knee
level, and pointed in front of you, and knees
are slightly apart. Lift your hands to your knees.
Inhale, and then exhale, tip your chin to your
chest and roll your head, neck and shoulders
up from the floor. Hold your shoulder blades
down in contact with the floor. Keep your
shoulders away from your ears and the
breastbone soft.

4 Grasp the outside of your right ankle with your
right hand, and hold onto your right knee with
your left hand. Exhale and extend your left leg
at an angle of 45 degrees to the floor, toes
pointing. Simultaneously draw the bent knee
closer to the chest. As you draw the knee back
towards your chest, the shin should remain
parallel to the floor, with the heel away from the
back of the thigh. Your extended leg, meanwhile,
pulls away from the shoulders and the shoulders
pull away from the extended leg in opposition,
to balance the movement. Hold for a few deep
breaths and then, on inhale, fold your left knee
back in towards your chest.

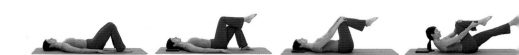

5 Now change hands and legs and on exhale repeat step 4 to extend the right leg. Repeat ten times, alternating legs.

reminders: Extend your leg as you exhale. The bottom tips of your shoulder blades should be in contact with the floor throughout. Keep the neutral pelvis throughout – no bulging stomach! The spine should not arch, so hold the back of your ribcage down and keep the tailbone down. Maintain a long, straight line from the breastbone to the pubic bone. Use your hands to help guide your leg straight back to you: one hand holds the outside of the ankle, or just above it, while the other holds the knee (see right), and your elbows remain open. Be careful not to rock from side to side; you should stay firmly planted.

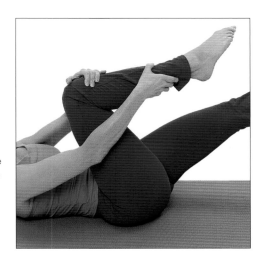

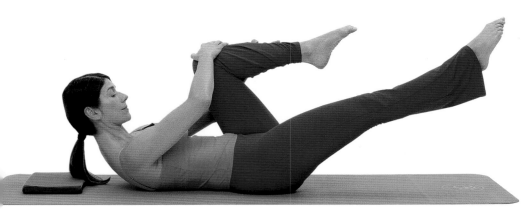

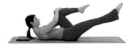

chiropractor's comments
Make sure you really feel your abdominal muscles squeezing and working. Pay attention to your lower spine so that it is nice and flat on the ground – do not arch!

open leg rocker prep

aims

to improve balance; to maintain a strong centre as the arms and legs move; and to lengthen the spine and stretch the legs.

chiropractor's comments

This is an excellent exercise for strengthening the quadriceps and stabilizing the shoulders. It is important to keep the spine lifted and strong while you are holding the pose.

1 Sit up tall with your legs stretched out in front of you. Draw your navel back to your spine to engage your deep abdominals.

2 Keeping your back straight and long, and looking forwards, open your knees until they are about a shoulder-width apart. Reach between your legs to take hold of your ankles.

3 Lift your feet just off the floor and lean back slightly onto the tailbone. The key to this exercise is learning exactly how far to tip your pelvis back and still hold strong. Inhale, lengthen your spine and prepare for the leg extension.

4 Exhale and extend your right leg up as high as you can, lifting up the chest, lower back and stomach as you do so. Don't collapse down into your lower back; keep pulling down your shoulder blades towards your waist and focus on lengthening the neck. Look straight ahead.

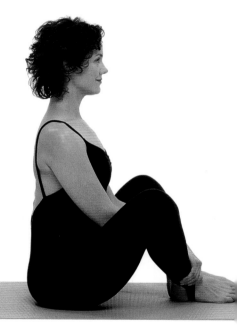

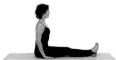

Inhale and bring your right leg back down to the starting position, with the feet just off the floor.

 Exhale and extend your left leg up as high as you can, lifting the chest, lower back and stomach – as you have just done with the right leg in step 4.

 Inhale and then release the left leg, letting it return to the starting position – with the feet just above the floor and holding the ankles with your hands.

 Now exhale, straighten both legs, and extend them in front of you in a 'V' shape, with your hands grasping your ankles. Keep your arms, legs and spine straight and drop your shoulders down and away from your ears. Repeat the entire sequence three times.

reminders: Keep your arms, legs and spine straight throughout. Lift out of the lower back and out of the stomach.

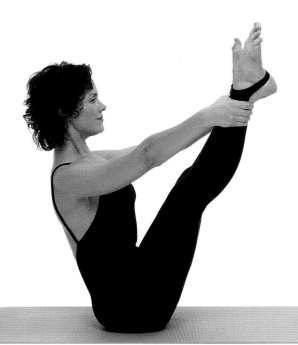

sitting spine twist

aims

to stretch the spine, the sides of the trunk and the hamstrings, while maintaining a strong aligned centre; to work the deep abdominals; and to introduce rotation.

1 Sit up straight with your legs stretched out in front of you, and as wide apart as is comfortable. If your legs feel tight and you find your pelvis tends to tip backwards, sit on a phone book, a rolled-up towel or a yoga block. Raise your arms out to the sides, just in front of the body line – just below shoulder level and parallel to the floor, with your palms facing the floor. Inhale, lengthen your spine and pull your shoulder blades down.

2 Exhale, draw your navel to your spine and engage as you twist round to the right, keeping your arms as wide apart as in step 1. Look to the right. Keep your pelvis and legs absolutely still, as if your lower body is set in cement. The twist is initiated by your stomach muscles, so move the left side of your stomach to the right and then let the upper body follow, rather than pulling on the shoulders.

3 Inhale and come back to the centre starting position. Keep your spine lengthened and your shoulder blades down.

4 Repeat the twist to the left side, keeping your pelvis and legs still and twisting with your stomach muscles, allowing your upper body to follow. Now alternate sides to twist a further five times on each side.

reminders: This should be a relaxed, smooth movement, without tension.

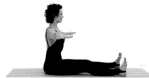
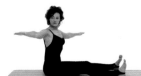
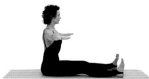

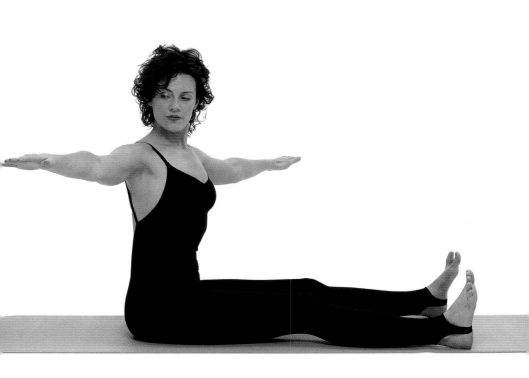

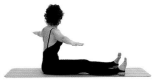

chiropractor's comments

This is an excellent exercise for introducing gentle rotation through your lower spine. Keep lifted and alive through your abdominal and pelvic muscles. As you work in this pose you will feel a gentle stretch in your hamstrings.

side leg kicks ups & downs

aims

to maintain a strong, stable centre while making large, controlled leg movements, and to lengthen from that centre; to strengthen, lengthen and tone the hips, buttocks and outer thighs; and to stretch and tone the inner thighs.

1 Lie on your side in alignment. Your spine should be along the back edge of the mat, while your feet are at the front edge. Keep legs together and feet flexed. Turn out the top of your leg so that your knee faces the ceiling and point your toes. Keep one hip directly on top of the other. Inhale to lengthen the spine and prepare.

2 Exhale, draw your navel to your spine as you engage, and kick your top leg up to the ceiling without changing the position of your hips. Keep your head in line with your spine as you kick, and don't let your upper body come out of alignment.

3 Inhale, and slowly lower your leg, working with the resistance. As you do so, stretch out your leg, making it as long as possible. Return to the starting position and repeat ten times. Then change sides, lying on the opposite hip, to work the other leg.

reminders: The top leg remains turned out throughout, while the bottom leg remains in parallel on the floor. Engage the buttocks to help to rotate the leg. Nothing moves but the kicking leg – hold stable in your centre.

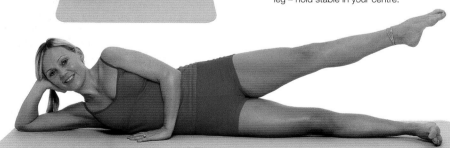

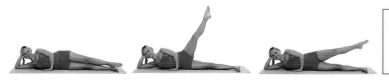

chiropractor's comments

Excellent for strengthening the lateral thigh, buttocks and lateral stabilizers of the knee.

dart

aims

to strengthen the back of the body and lengthen the spine; to strengthen and stabilize the shoulders, and work the deep neck muscles; to build strength in the muscles that stabilize the pelvis.

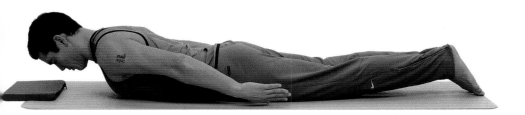

1 Lie face-down on the floor, and position a thin pillow on which to rest your forehead. Lie in correct alignment, as if there's a tennis ball under your belly button, so that your stomach doesn't push into the floor – this way your lower back will remain long. Your arms should be down at your sides and your legs should be squeezing together with your toes pointed. Lengthen the neck and look at the floor. Inhale, lengthen your spine and prepare.

2 Exhale and engage the pelvic floor as you lift your upper body off the floor, pulling the shoulder blades down towards your waist and sending your arms down and away towards your feet. Your neck pulls away from your shoulders, and your shoulders pull away from your head, lengthening the neck. Keep looking at the floor – don't lift your head as this will shorten the neck. Keep squeezing your inner thighs and keep your feet on the floor. Feel your body lengthen. Then inhale and release to come down. Repeat five times.

reminders: Keep your stomach hollow and lifted away from the floor. The inner thighs and buttocks should remain engaged throughout.

> **chiropractor's comments**
> This is a great exercise for strengthening the large erector spinae muscles of the spine – the main support structure of your back. Do not overarch the spine and try to stay long and lifted through your neck and shoulders.

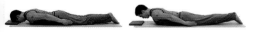

full swan dive

aims

to stretch and strengthen all the muscles in the back of the body, and to have fun!

1 Lie on your stomach with your palms directly under your shoulders and pressing into the mat. Your legs should be hip-width apart. Lengthen them out and away from your hips; point your toes, and press them down into the mat. Engage the backs of the legs and the buttocks.

2 Inhale as you draw your navel back to the spine and engage your back muscles. Pull your shoulder blades down and straighten your arms to lift your upper body off the floor, keeping your neck long. Exhale, and lower your body back down to the mat. Repeat five times to warm up.

chiropractor's comments

The full swan dive is the ultimate back strengthener for your spinal muscles. It is a difficult pose; if you feel any discomfort or pain in your lower back, please stop immediately. If you lift the head away from the pelvis, it will help to elongate and stretch the spine. Feel the buttocks and the back come alive with energy.

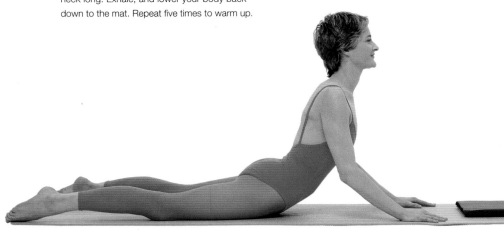

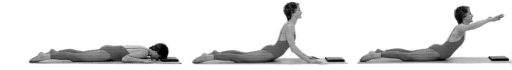

3 As you stretch up for the sixth time, lifting your chest, with your neck long and your shoulders down, hold your upper body stable and raise your hands out in a 'V' in front of you.

4 Rock forwards like a see-saw, lifting your legs up high behind you as your chest drops down to the floor. Your arms should still be out in front of you, with the palms down.

5 Use the momentum you've created to swing your upper body back up high to the ceiling, and then continue to rock back and forth. Inhale as you dive forwards and exhale as you come back, trying to make each dive larger than its predecessor. Repeat five times.

reminders: Maintain a strong, solid body as you rock back and forth. Breathe well and do not throw your head back. Keep your head in line with your arms as much as possible, lifting your chest and lengthening the back of your neck, but remember to keep your shoulders down. Your arms and momentum will help the rocking movement, but the main work should be done by the contracting muscles in your back.

kneeling side kick

aims

to improve alignment; to improve balance and coordination; and to work the waist, open the hips and build core strength.

1 Kneel up on a mat, with your knees hip-width apart, and your arms hanging loosely by your sides, with your shoulders down.

2 Place your right hand down on the mat under your right shoulder. Bring your left hand up so that it is behind your head, with your elbow bent and pointing up to the sky.

3 Extend your left leg along the mat in line with your body so that your left foot forms a straight line with your right knee and right hand.

4 Exhale. Lift your outstretched leg off the mat, keeping it in line with the body. Keep your hips pushed forwards, your chest open and the lifted elbow reaching up. Look straight ahead. You should feel as if you are pressed between two plates of glass, with your entire body in the same plane.

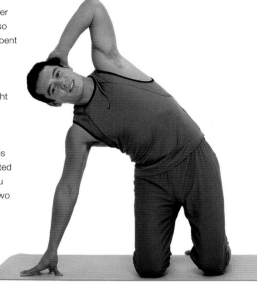

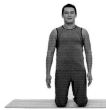

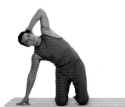

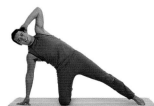

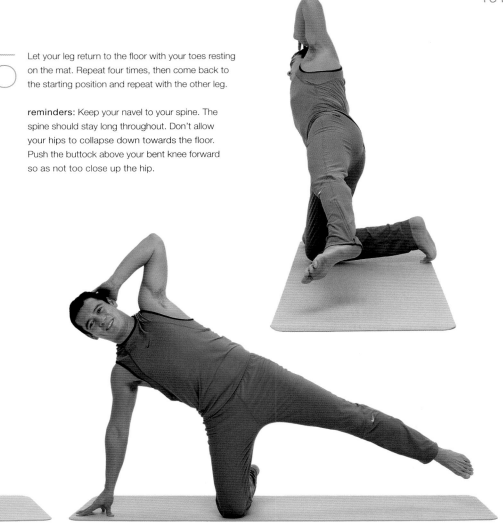

5　Let your leg return to the floor with your toes resting on the mat. Repeat four times, then come back to the starting position and repeat with the other leg.

reminders: Keep your navel to your spine. The spine should stay long throughout. Don't allow your hips to collapse down towards the floor. Push the buttock above your bent knee forward so as not too close up the hip.

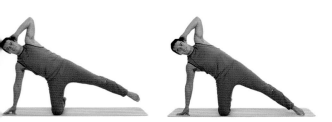

chiropractor's comments

A maximal exercise for developing core stabilization and a strong lower back, this exercise primarily targets the transverse abdominals, deep back muscles and the buttocks.

rolling like a ball

aims

to learn control; to build strong abdominals; and to massage and improve the flexibility of the spine.

1 Sit near the front of the mat with your knees bent and your arms round your knees so that you hold your knees with your hands. Look straight ahead.

2 Now tuck your chin into your chest and, staying balanced on your tailbone, lift your feet off the floor, one leg at a time.

3 When you have both feet off the floor, balance on your tailbone with your pelvis tilted slightly backwards. Inhale and prepare to roll.

4 Exhale and roll backwards, drawing your knees closer to your nose and pressing each vertebra down into the floor as you roll. Make sure you sink your navel deep into your spine and keep your stomach hollow.

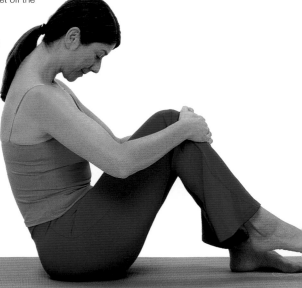

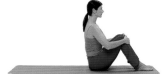

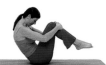

5 Inhale and roll back up to a sitting position. Stay balanced, pause and exhale, without letting your feet touch the floor. Then roll back down again as in step 4. Repeat five full rolls.

reminders: Keep your shoulders down, away from your ears. Don't throw your head back and don't roll back onto your neck. Keep tucked in tightly with your abdominals engaged throughout.

chiropractor's comments

If you have a spine- or disc-related problem please consult your doctor before embarking on this exercise, and it is not recommended if you have scoliosis or osteoporosis. The rolling sequence is a great stretch for relaxing and opening the segmental joints of the lumbar spine and giving the buttocks a gentle stretch. Focus on being very controlled in your movement and do not overload the lower neck.

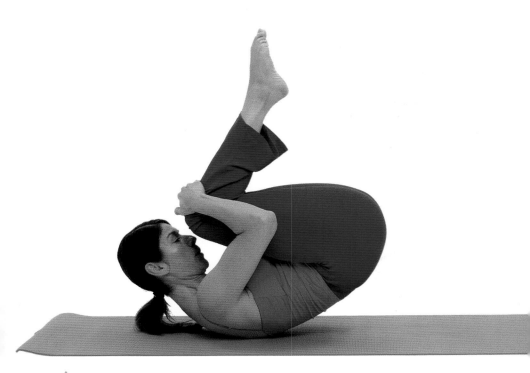

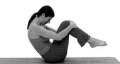

cat twist

aims

to develop coordination; to strengthen the back; to open the spine, chest and shoulders; and to rotate the spine and relax the muscles of the upper back.

> **chiropractor's comments**
> This is a great exercise because it promotes a healthy and flexible upper body. It works by releasing and stretching the shoulders and the upper thoracic spine – an area of the spine that can normally be very stiff and restricted.

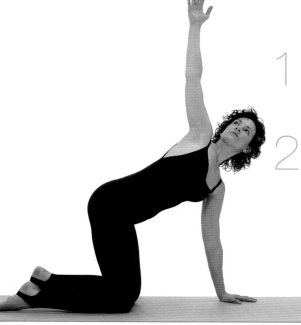

1 Kneel on your hands and knees, with your hands directly beneath your shoulders and your knees directly under your hips. Keep your neck and spine long and your head in line with your spine. Look down at the floor.

2 Inhale and, without locking your elbow, fix your left arm strongly on the mat as you swing your right arm up to the sky, reaching up with your fingertips, with the palm open. Turn your head to look up at your hand but keep the lower body still – only the upper body moves.

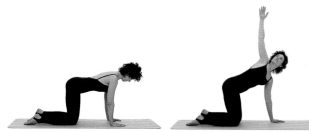
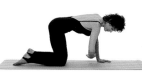

3 Exhale as you curl the right arm back down and slide it under your body, sliding it along the floor in a line just behind your supporting left hand.

4 Bend your left elbow and drop your head and right shoulder down onto the mat to complete the stretch. Inhale and reverse the movement. Repeat five times on each side.

reminders: As you reach up to the ceiling, lift from the breastbone, so that your chest is open without any struggle in the arms or shoulders. Keep your arms long and straight without locking them at the elbows. Lift up from a firm base formed by the stabilizing hand on the floor, rather than letting yourself collapse down on the lower arm.

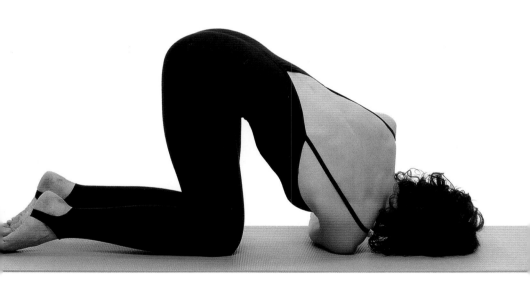

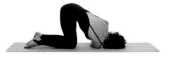

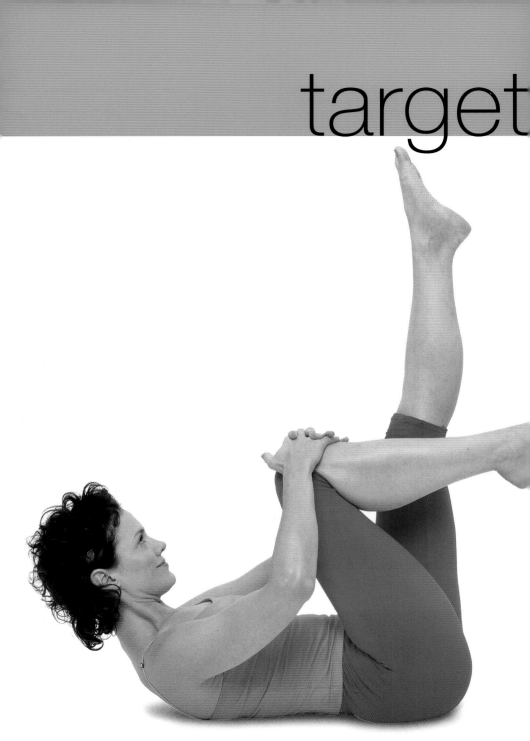

exercises

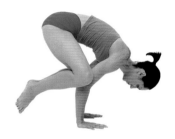

These three target exercises can be performed on their own or with a warm-up (see pages 24–37). A few minutes is all you need to do the energy-boost exercises, which will raise your energy levels – fast! Back ache is usually caused by poor posture and a lack of strength in the body's core muscles, and the back-strength programme works both the deep stabilizing and spinal muscles to help alleviate an existing condition or prevent a future problem. Stress is not just something in your head – it can bring about high blood pressure and emotional and physical exhaustion. The restorative destress exercises that follow can help to ease anxiety and promote an overall sense of balance.

Before performing this exercise, please complete **freestanding roll down** on page 70.

pole twist

aims

to build good core strength; to teach you to lead from the centre; to lengthen and to release tension in the spine; and to stabilize and twist the centre.

1 Stand in alignment with the pole resting on your shoulders and your arms wrapped around it (as shown). Inhale to prepare.

2 Exhale, engage and draw your navel to your spine. Twist to the right, initiating the move from your stomach, twisting the left part of your waist to the right, following with your upper body. Keep your hips still: there should be no movement below the waist. Look to the right.

3 Inhale and come back to the centre. Then repeat the movement to the left. Alternate sides, repeating the twist five times on each side.

reminders: Keep the alignment. Lengthen your neck and spine. Plant your feet firmly on the ground and don't move your hips.

> **chiropractor's comments**
> A gentle rotational exercise for the mid and lower spine. Feel the back with its segmental motion opening up between each joint.

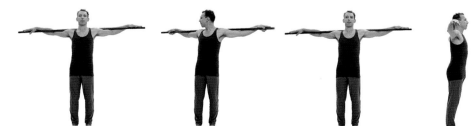

Before performing this exercise,
please complete **bridge** on page 117.

109

star

aims

to create and condition a stabilizing strength in all the muscles at the back
of the body; and to develop a strong centre from which to lengthen out.

chiropractor's comments
Excellent for deep back strength and core stability. This
is a tough exercise, so work on your strength level slowly.

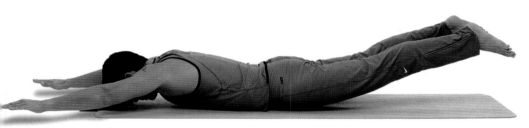

1   Lie face-down on the floor with your forehead
    resting on a thin pillow. Your feet should be slightly
    wider than hip-width apart and arms just wider
    than shoulder-width apart. Imagine you have a
    tennis ball under your belly button. Don't push
    your stomach into the floor! Inhale to prepare.

2   Exhale, engage deeply and draw your navel to
    your spine. Lift your right leg and left arm about
    13 cm (5 in) off the floor and lengthen them. Avoid
    pushing your stomach into the floor, and your
    forehead should be barely lifted off the pillow. As
    your head pulls away from your shoulders and your
    shoulders pull away from your head, keep your
    neck long. Inhale and relax back down to the floor.
    Alternate sides, repeating five times on each side.

3   Inhale to prepare, then exhale and engage, your
    navel drawn to your spine. Lift both arms and
    both legs off the floor. Lengthen both your arms
    and legs, remembering to keep your stomach
    lifted and your neck long, as above.

4   Now inhale and relax down again. Exhale and
    then repeat five times.

    reminders: Keep your arm away from your ear
    as you lift it, so that your shoulders remain low and
    stable. Keep your hip bones down on the floor.

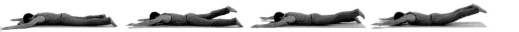

locust

aims

to open and lengthen the front of the body, in order to release the back, and to strengthen every muscle in the back of the body!

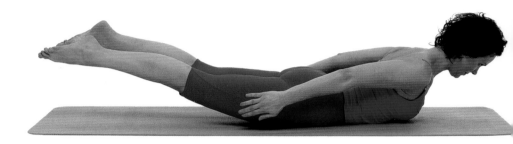

1 Lie face-down with your forehead resting on the floor, your arms down at your sides, and your palms facing your thighs. Your legs should be slightly apart and your stomach is lifted off the floor slightly. Inhale to prepare.

2 Exhale, engage and draw your navel to your spine as you lift your chest, thighs and feet off the floor. Feel a pull through your toes as you stretch your legs away from your hips, long and straight. Reach further behind you with your arms and pull your shoulder blades down towards your waist, pulling your fingertips away from your wrists. Reach even further with your arms to lift your chest higher. Look slightly forward, without pulling your head up and straining your neck. Relax down and repeat three times.

variation: Use this modified pose if you have any lower back pain. Lie face-down and place your palms flat beside your chest, elbows bent and shoulder blades down. Press firmly into the floor and lift your head and chest, pulling the chest forward and your legs away from hips as you lift.

reminders: Engage strongly in the buttocks and thighs. Drop the shoulders down towards your waist and away from your ears. The legs should pull away from the hips as the chest pulls forward away from them to work the opposition.

> **chiropractor's comments**
> During the exercise, concentrate on the strength of the buttocks and thighs to help support the lumbar spine (lower back). The pose is a difficult one to accomplish.

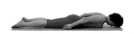

variation

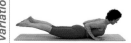

bow

aims

to work all the muscles in the back of the body, simultaneously opening and stretching the front of the body, and to energize!

1 Lie face-down on the floor with your arms at your sides, elbows tucked near the ribs and palms flat on the floor. The forehead rests on the floor and legs stretch straight out behind you.

2 Bend both legs in towards the buttocks, keeping knees and feet at hip-width apart. Grab the ankles from the outside with your thumbs pointing down to the floor.

3 Inhale, pull on your ankles and lift your head, chest and thighs off the floor. Take your shoulders back and keep your arms straight. Lift in the front of your body. Now lift your legs higher so that your torso pushes forward and your legs resist, pulling up and back.

reminders: Look forward, maintain a strong grip on your ankles and keep lifting the legs higher.

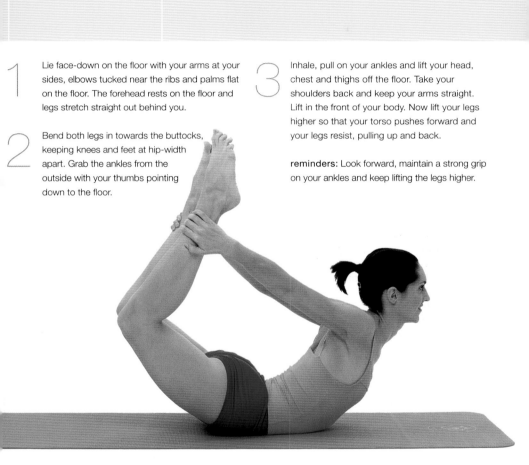

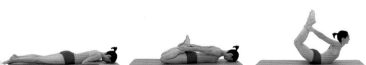

chiropractor's comments
Please consult your doctor if you have a history of spinal or disc-related injury.

crescent lunge

aims

to build strength in the entire body, and to connect the strength of the lower body, upper body and central core; to open up the upper body and hips; and to build a flowing, connected sequence.

chiropractor's comments

Builds coordination and strength in the thighs. Feel the opening of the anterior thigh muscle when the leg is back.

1 Start off in the dog pose (see steps 1–3 on page 74).

2 From dog pose, exhale and step your right foot forwards between your hands, finishing with your knee bent, so that your thigh is parallel to the floor. Press down on the ball of your left foot, lifting the heel off the floor, and pushing out through the heel. Now lift the back of your left thigh, and connect down the back of your left leg from buttock to heel. Both your hips and feet should be squarely to the front throughout.

3 Inhale and sweep the arms up from the sides to shoulder level, lifting the torso into an upright position as you stabilize the lower body.

4 Continue this sweeping movement upwards so that your hands finish over your head, with your arms straight and parallel, palms facing. Drop your shoulder blades down, away from your ears.

Lengthen the spine, lift the chest, keeping your ribcage back in a straight line above the hips. Pull your tailbone down and lift the top of your head. The spine is long; the stomach lifts up and away from your front thigh; and the left hip pulls back while the right stays forward, keeping the hips square. Remember to keep the back leg active and strong. Look straight ahead. Now reverse back through this sequence to return to dog pose and then repeat on the other side.

reminders: The thigh and shin of your front leg should form a right angle at the knee. Lift your arms higher and higher! Your feet should be parallel, about 10 cm (4 in) apart.

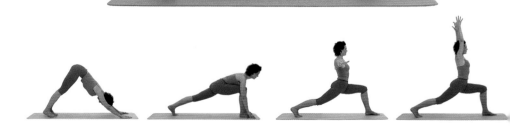

warrior 2

aims

to build strength in the entire body and connect the strength of lower body, core and upper body; to achieve an open, strong pose; to open the hips; and to strengthen and tone the buttocks, thighs, shoulders, arms, abdominals and deep spinal muscles.

chiropractor's comments
This builds strength in your thigh muscles while opening and stretching tight hip flexors. Keep strong and lifted through your lumbar spine (lower back).

1 Standing tall, extend your arms to the sides at shoulder level and step your feet wide apart so that they are directly beneath your fingertips and parallel, hips and feet facing the front.

2 Now turn out your left foot so that it points directly to the left, and allow the right heel to rotate by about 15 degrees. Pull up on the knees of both legs to engage the legs strongly. Push your back foot firmly into the floor as you lunge to the left, bending your left knee to form a right angle, with your thigh parallel to the floor. Draw your right arm back a little so that your torso leans back slightly, but keep your weight equally distributed on both legs. Pull the shoulder blades down towards your waist, and reach through the middle finger on both hands, pulling your arms in opposite directions. Fingertip to fingertip, the stretch through your wide open arms is long. Focus on the middle finger of your front hand. Hold for 30 seconds, and then reverse back to the starting position. Repeat on the other side.

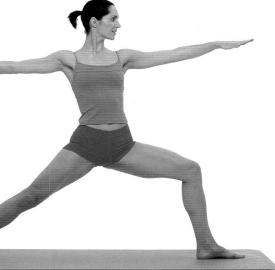

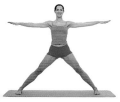 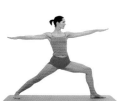

reminders: Stretch the mat apart with your feet. Lift your stomach, spine and chest, but keep your shoulders down. Your front thigh is low, parallel to the floor.

side-plank against the wall

aims

to make all the muscles work together; to provide the strength necessary to support your body weight; and to get the entire body working!

chiropractor's comments

One of the best lower back stability exercises! Feel your lower back muscles working hard and keep lifted through your hips.

1 With your back to a wall, kneel down on your hands and knees so that your feet are about 30cm (12 in) away from the wall.

2 Extend your right leg back to the wall. Curl your toes under and push your heel back into the wall as you straighten the leg.

3 Now extend your left leg back, curling your toes under and pushing your heel back into the wall as you straighten the leg. As you push back, feel the connection of the strength in your legs, buttocks, deep abdominals, spine and shoulders. Keep your hips lifted, but slightly lower than your shoulders, and keep your shoulders strong and high. Look down at the floor. You are now in the plank pose.

4 Make sure your feet are touching and then lift your right hand off the floor and rotate your body back, rolling onto the side of your left foot. Open your chest and reach up to the sky with your right hand. Keep your supporting arm strong by ensuring that your left hand is directly under your shoulder. Push your feet into the wall to stabilize, and push the buttocks forwards as you pull your tailbone away from your shoulders. Roll your shoulders and chest back. Keep your neck long, and your chin up. If you can look up at your right hand, do so. Check your alignment, imagining you are pressed between two plates of glass. Hold for 30 seconds, and then reverse out. Repeat on the other side.

reminders: Keep your hips high and your chest open so that you create a long stretch from hand to hand.

mountain pose to standing forward bend

aims

to warm up the body, and make contact with the body and the breath; to build core strength; to open the upper body; to stretch and strengthen the spine and strengthen and lengthen the legs; and to learn the beginning of the sun salutation sequence.

chiropractor's comments

Proceed if you feel no adherent strain on the lower back or hamstrings. Use the alternate bent knee variation if the other one seems too difficult – it will help you to prevent injury.

1 Stand in mountain pose with your arms above your head and your palms together (see page 26). Lift the chest and inhale.

2 Now exhale and sweep forward and down with a straight spine, hinged at the hips, and lengthening from the base of the spine. Sweep your arms down sideways, taking the fingertips to the floor, or holding onto your ankles. Release your head from the shoulders so it hangs freely, with your neck relaxed. Your hips should be directly above your heels. Press your chest towards the thighs. Keep your legs straight, but if you feel any strain, bend the knees. Reverse and repeat five times.

variations: Bending your knees and placing your hands on the floor with your head slightly raised will relieve strain on your spine. Alternatively, modify the stretch by bending forward with your knees bent and resting your elbows on your thighs. This allows you to lengthen your spine and feel stable without strain – and allows your body to be supported by your thighs. Alternatively, use a chair to support the forward bend. Hold the pose for 30 seconds.

reminders: Press down evenly on both feet so that you are balanced. Don't sway as you bend and come back up. If you do start to sway, take your feet further apart to stabilize yourself. Maintain alignment, so that your hips are directly over your thighs, knees, calves, ankles and feet. Soften and draw in your stomach to lengthen the spine.

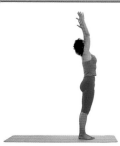

variations

the crow

aims

to build upper body, deep abdominal and deep core strength; to develop balance; and to develop a sense of lightness as your feet lift off the floor.

1 Squat down on the floor, with your feet shoulder-width apart and your arms between your knees.

2 Press your hands onto the floor just in front of your feet, with fingers forwards. Lift your hips up high and lean forwards, opening your knees slightly and pressing your elbows against the inside of your knees. Let your hips lift even higher as you tip your head down to the floor and rock forwards. Now, keeping your hips high and engaging your deep abdominals strongly to keep your stomach lifted, lift your feet off the floor in a little hop.

3 Rock backwards again to reverse the movement, until your feet come back down and then your hands come slightly off the floor, as in step 1. Now have a bit of fun and rock backwards and forwards to get a sense of balance and to understand how, if the whole body works together, it is easy to lift your entire body weight in a relaxed way.

> **chiropractor's comments**
> Great for building strength, stability and coordination into the shoulder girdle muscles. Use caution or avoid entirely if you have a history of wrist- or shoulder-related problems.

4 Now, as you lean forwards again, slowly peel your right foot off the floor to find your balance before you lift up your left foot.

5 Lift your left foot to balance on your hands. Keep toes pointed and touching, with feet level with your knees. Lift hips higher, draw your navel back to the spine, and keep your stomach in. Engage every muscle and look up, if possible.

reminders: Keep your back rounded and lean forwards.

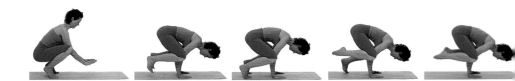

bridge

aims

to open the front of the body; to tone the buttocks and thighs; to release the lower back; to improve breathing; to connect the mind and body with breath; and to relax the mind.

1 Lie on your back with your feet parallel, hip-width apart and placed close to your buttocks. Your arms should be down at your sides, close to your hips, palms facing the floor.

chiropractor's comments
This is excellent for developing buttock strength and core stability, which is essential for a healthy lower back.

2 Inhale, press your feet down firmly and lift your hips high to rest on your shoulders. Press your upper arms down into the floor. Keep your knees hip-width apart and your feet parallel. Look at your nose, exhale and then reverse back down to the floor. Repeat ten times. This is part of a dynamic breathing and movement sequence, so keep moving as you inhale on rising up and exhale on coming down. Repeat ten times.

reminders: Your feet should be parallel and hip-width apart. If this is uncomfortable, place your feet wider apart, still parallel to each other.

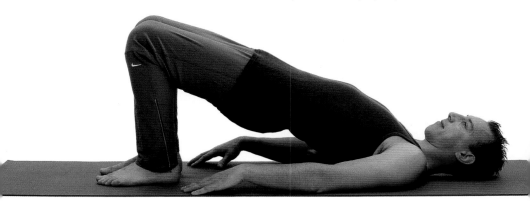

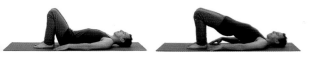

supported child's pose

aims

to relax and release all the muscles of the body; to slow down the heart rate; to link breath and body; and to direct the focus inwards.

1 Roll three neatly piled blankets to form a bolster or, alternatively, use a ready-made bolster.

2 Kneel at the end of your bolster. Point your toes so that the tops of your feet are flat on the floor. Rest your hips on your heels, and place your hands lightly on your thighs. Your spine should be long and straight.

3 Your big toes should be touching while your knees are wide, one on each side of the bolster.

4 Keep your spine straight and long as you walk your hands forward until your entire torso rests on the bolster, from pelvis to head. The front of the body is supported, so the back muscles can lengthen and spread. Let go of all tension. Drop deeper into the bolster and drape your arms loosely around it. If possible, allow your hips to rest on your heels. Turn your head to one side for two minutes and then to the other side for a further two minutes. Relax the breath.

reminders: Breathe freely and deeply – hear the sound of the breath deep inside you. Draw your focus inwards.

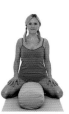

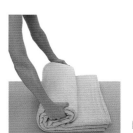
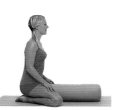
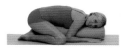

legs up the wall with blankets

aims

to cleanse the lower limbs and nourish the upper body, neck and head by the downward flow of blood; to improve concentration; to alleviate fatigue and varicose veins; and to stretch the spine, the front of the body and hamstrings. The benefits of inversion are received without effort as you are supported.

chiropractor's comments
This leg stretch is great for relieving tension in the legs, while gently stretching the hamstrings.

1 Place a pile of folded blankets against the wall. Sit sideways to the wall at the edge of the blankets, with your hips touching the wall and your knees tucked into your chest.

2 Using your left arm for support, lie down so that your left hip is on the blankets and both buttocks are against the wall.

3 Now turn over onto your back so that you are lying with your hips and lower back supported by blankets, your tailbone touching the wall and your head on the floor. Keep your hips square.

4 Press your shoulders down into the floor and lift your chest. Your arms rest on the floor, away from your body, with the palms face-up. Extend legs up the wall. With your legs together and straight, press lightly against the wall with feet flexed, as if you were standing on the floor. Your hips should stay as close to the wall as possible; if straightening your legs is difficult, move your hips away from the wall. Close your eyes, breathe comfortably and hold for one to three minutes. Come down slowly by bending your knees and rolling onto your side.

reminders: You can take your hips further away from the wall if you find this pose uncomfortable.

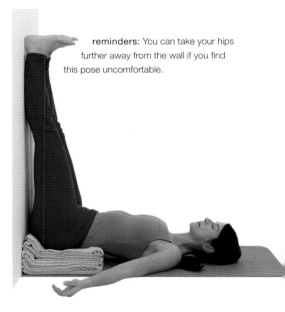

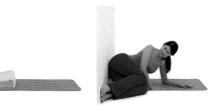
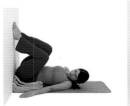
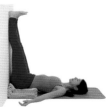

shoulderstand at the wall

aims

to calm the mind and refresh the body; and to soothe and nourish the entire body with the benefits of an inversion posture without effort, as you are supported by a wall.

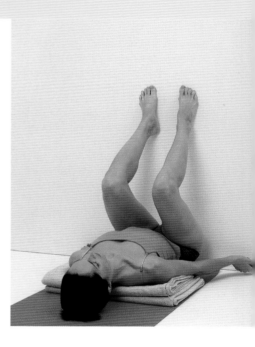

1 Place three folded blankets exactly above each other in a neat pile on the floor about 25 cm (10 in) away from a wall.

2 Lie near the wall on the edge of the blankets, with hips touching the wall, knees tucked into the chest and your right shoulder on the blanket.

3 Lie back so the shoulders rest on the blankets' top edge. The neck and hips are on the floor. Bring your knees to your chest and your feet to the wall.

4 Lift your hips, press your shoulders to the floor and walk your feet up the wall. Support your back by bringing your hands to your hips. Keep drawing your elbows closer and pull your shoulder blades towards each other. As legs straighten, move your hands down. Do not arch your back or lift your ribs too high. Look at your chest. Steady the body, relax your breathing and hold for two minutes. Reverse the steps to come back down – slowly.

variation: Come up as in step 4 but do not straighten your legs.

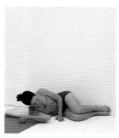
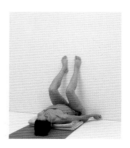
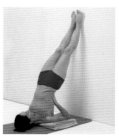

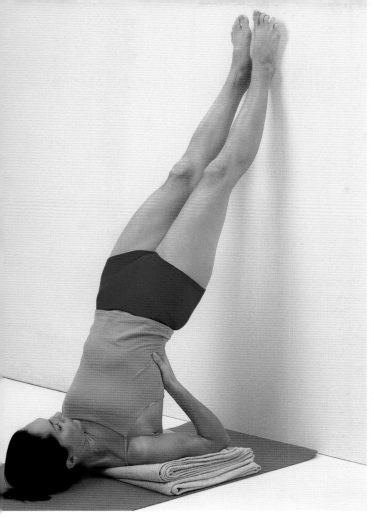

chiropractor's comments

Skip this exercise if you suffer from neck or lower back problems – and especially if you have a history of whiplash. If you feel pain in the cervical spine (neck), stop the exercise immediately. Make sure that you are tightening your buttocks and abdominals to support the pelvis and lower back. Your weight should be distributed equally on both shoulders.

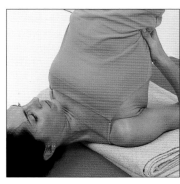

variation

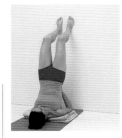

reminders: Do not stay in this pose if you feel pressure in the head, eyes, ears or throat. Your inner armpits open outwards as the outer edges of shoulders push down into the floor. You are resting on the outside upper edges of the shoulders, not the neck. Allow a gap between your chin and chest.

half-plough with legs to the wall

aims

to stretch the entire back and soothe the nervous system.

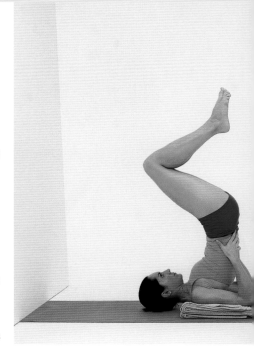

1
Sit up straight, with your legs outstretched and your feet touching the wall. Mark the position of your hip bones with a yoga brick on the floor.

2
Fold three blankets (see shoulderstand, pages 120–1) and place the front edge level with the yoga brick. Place another folded blanket below.

3
Lie back with the top of your shoulders on the edge of the blankets. The head rests on the floor; the neck is not supported by the blankets. Arms are at your sides.

4
Now, engaging your deep abdominal muscles, rock your hips forward and bring your knees to your chest.

5
Lift your hips off the floor and support your hips by placing your hands at your waist and pressing your elbows down into the floor. Bring your elbows and shoulder blades closer together and press your shoulders into the floor to lift the spine higher. Walk your hands down your spine towards the shoulder blades to lift your body even higher. Bring your ribcage forward. Look at your chest.

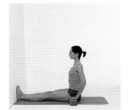
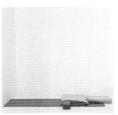
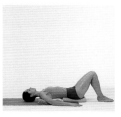
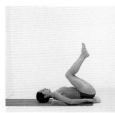

6 Now, holding steady in the entire body, slowly take one leg at a time to the wall. Rest the soles of your feet on the wall behind you.

7 Walk your feet down the wall until they are level with your hips so that the hips are above your shoulders and the heels are level with your hips. Lift up the front of your body and lengthen up the

sides. Open the back of the legs to lift the back of the thighs. Lift up your pubic bone, and push your hips backwards and your ribcage forwards.

reminders: Do not turn your head to either side while in the plough or you could strain your neck. Focus on keeping both the front of the body and the spine lifted.

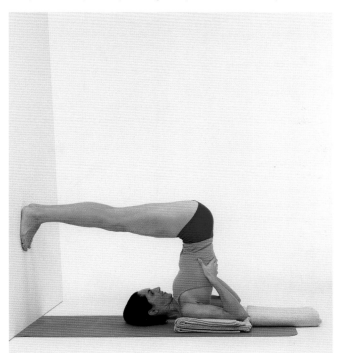

chiropractor's comments

Please do not do this exercise if you suffer from neck or lower back problems. It is essential to keep the pelvis and lower back strong and lifted. You should be able to feel the tightness release in your back as you become comfortable and stationary in the pose.

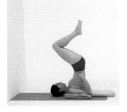
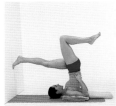
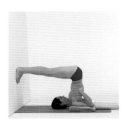

reclined cobbler pose

aims

to soothe the nervous system and relax the lower back and hips while stretching the muscles of the inner thighs.

1 Sit upright and place a bolster behind you. Press your buttocks against the flat end. (You can use flat edge of three rolled blankets, as described on page 118.) Place a small pillow at the top edge of the bolster to rest your head on.

2 Now bend your knees and open them out to the sides, bringing your feet up close to your hips, soles together. As you tuck your buttocks under, lie back on the bolster, flattening out the curve of your lower back to the bolster. Relax and lie all the way back, resting your head on the pillow. Your arms are about 20 cm (8 in) away from your body, with the elbows softly bent and the palms

> **chiropractor's comments**
> Great for opening the pelvis, and stretching the hip flexors and the medial thigh muscles – areas that are normally very tight if you sit all day. Feel a gentle stretch through your spine and be careful not to overarch.

facing up. Slide your shoulder blades down towards the waist so that the front of the body is wide open. Allow your stomach to drop. Close your eyes and relax your breathing.

reminders: If your lower back feels strained in this pose, move the bolster further away from your hips. As your knees are unsupported when they are wide open, prop them up with pillows or a chair if you feel any pain in your hips or thighs.

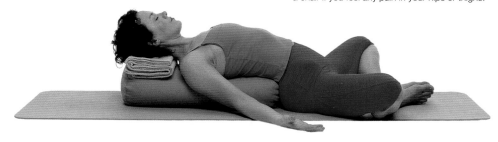

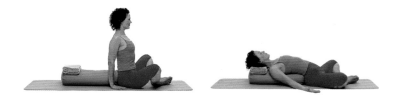

corpse

aims

to end with the deepest rest of all, taking you into a slightly meditative state, and to learn to fully surrender! Don't worry if you fall asleep.

1 Lie on your back with your legs out straight and hip-width apart. Let your knees and feet roll out to each side. Rest your arms on the floor about 30 cm (12 in) away from your body, palms facing up. Roll your shoulder blades towards each other to open your chest. Lengthen the spine and make contact with the floor. Drop down deeper into it, close your eyes and relax every bit of your body – from feet to head – as you focus on each area in turn and observe it, and then drop down and release. Listen to your heartbeat, feel the pulse in your solar plexus and listen to your breathing. Rest here for five minutes.

reminders: Place a blanket or thin pillow beneath your head if this feels more comfortable.

chiropractor's comments

Relax your body into this restful state. Become aware of how your hips, shoulders and spine feel in relation to the rest of your body. Feel the circulation of air into your lung as it expands and stretches your ribs and chest wall. Enjoy the pose.

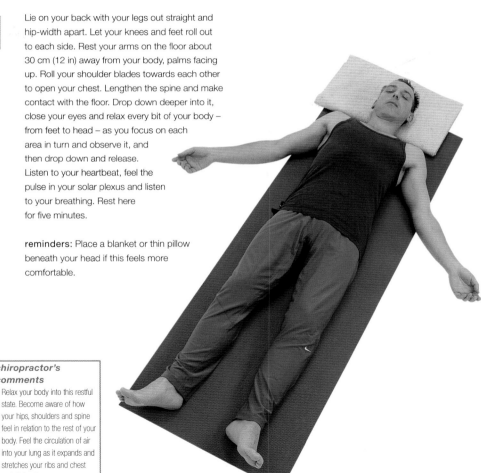

index

Figures in italics indicate captions.

resources
glossary

abdominal muscles –
a group of four muscles
which make up the
abdominal wall.
a. Rectus abdominis – the
midline stomach muscle
that originates from the
pubic bone to the cartilage
of the fifth to seventh ribs.
b. Oblique abdominals
(external and internal) –
these lay diagonally to the
rectus abdominis. They are
important muscles for
lateral strength of the
lumbar spine.
c. Transverse abdominis –
supports your lumbar spine
and abdominal wall.

cervical spine – the top
seven vertebrae of the spine
that make up the bony axis
of the neck.

coccygeal spine – the
four vertebrae comprising
the triangular coccyx at
the bottom of the spine.

core muscles – comprises
the transverse abdominis,
the pelvic floor muscles
and the deep back
muscles (multifidus). Forms
the support structure of
the lower back, giving a
girdle of strength.

extensors – muscles that
extend or stretch an arm,
leg or other body part.

flexors – muscles that
contract to bend a joint
or limb.

lumbar spine – the five
vertebrae in the lower back
below the thoracic spine.

rotator cuff muscles –
a group of four muscles
(teres minor, subscapularis,
supraspinatus and
infraspinatus) that provide
the shoulder joints with
stability.

sacral spine, or sacrum – the large triangular bone made up of the five fused vertebrae below the lumbar spine.

thoracic spine – the twelve vertebrae directly between the cervical spine and the lumbar spine.

torsion – the act of twisting or the state of being twisted.

further reading

Ashtanga Yoga, The Practice Manual, David Swenson, Ashtanga Yoga Productions, 1999.

Awakening the Spine, Vanda Scaravelli, Aquarian, 1991.

The Body Control Pilates Back Book, Lynne Robinson, Helge Fisher and Paul Massey, Macmillan, 2002.

The Anatomy Coloring Book, Wynn Kapit and Lawrence M Elson, 3rd edn, Benjamin/ Cummings, 2001.

Anatomy of Movement, Blandine Calais-Germain, Eastland Press, 1993.

The Bhagavad Gita, Three Rivers Press, 2002. (Various translations are available.)

Cleanse and Purify Thyself Book One: The Cleanse and *Book Two: Secrets of Radiant Health and Energy*, Richard Anderson, Christobe Publishing, 2000.

Dynamic Alignment Through Imagery, Eric Franklin, Human Kinetics, 1997.

The Eight Human Talents, Kaur Khalsa Gurmukh and Cathryn Michon, Harper Resource, 2001.

The Heart of Yoga: Developing a Personal Practice, TKV Desikachar, Inner Traditions, 1995. (www.gotoit.com)

Journey into Power, How to Sculpt Your Ideal Body, Free Your True Self and Transform Your Life with Yoga, Baron Baptiste and Richard Corman (photographer), Fireside, 2002.

Light on Yoga, BKS Iyengar and Yehudi Menuhin, revised edn, Schocken Books, 1995. First published by George Allen & Unwin Ltd, 1966.

The Official Body Control Pilates Manual, Lynne Robinson, Helge Fisher, Jacqeline Knox, Gordon Thomson, et al, Pan–Macmillan, 2000.

The Pilates Body: The Ultimate At-Home Guide to Strengthening, Lengthening and Toning Your Body without Machines, Brooke Siler, Bantam Doubleday Dell, 2000.

Pilates, Return to Life through Contrololgy, Joseph H Pilates and William John Miller, Christopher Publishing, 1998.

Something Good for A Change... random notes on peace thru living, Wavy Gravy, St Martin's Press, 1992.

Super Power Breathing: For Super Energy, High Health and Longevity, Patricia Bragg, re-issued edn, Health Science, 1999.

The Art of Living: Vipassana Meditation as taught by S N Goenka, William Hart, Harper San Francisco, 1987.

Tao Te Ching: A New English Version, trans. Stephen Mitchell, Perennial, 1992.

Yoga... A Gem for Women, Geeta S Iyengar, Timeless Books, 1991.

Yoga for You, Indra Devi, David Lifszyc, Fundacion Indra Devi, Gibbs Smith Publisher, 2002.

Yoga, The Iyengar Way, Silva Mehta, Mira Mehta and Shyam Mehta, Alfred A Knopf, New York, 1990.

Yoga, Mastering the Basics, Sandra Anderson and Rolf Sovik, Himalayan Institute Press, 2002.

Yoga, The Path to Holistic Health, BKS Iyengar, DK Publishing, 2001.

Yoga, The Poetry of the Body, Rodney Yee, Nina Zolotow and Michel Venera (photographer), St Martin's Press, 2002.

useful addresses

Jill Everett
Flow Studio
AGL Metropolitan
Wharf, Wapping Wall
London E1W 3SS
tele: 0207 709 7234
www.flowstudio.co.uk
jillneverett@hotmail.com

Dr Jennifer Golay Bengston
Doctor of Chiropractic
9A Wilbraham Place
London SW1X 9AE
tele: 0207 730 3031

Bridget Woods-Kramer
Yoga Ltd
The Old Chapel
St Clements Street
Truro, Cornwall
tele: 0187 232 1111
www.omshop.com

websites

www.bheka.com
yoga props, mats and equipment (USA)

www.bksiyengaryoga.com
Iyengar teachers directory

www.bodycontrol.co.uk
Body Control Pilates teachers directory

www.omshop.com
yoga props, mats and equipment (UK/Europe)

www.pilatesfoundation.com
Pilates Foundation teachers directory

www.pilates-studio.com
The Pilates Studio teachers directory

www.stottpilates.com
Stott Pilates teachers directory

www.viniyoga.com
Vini yoga teachers directory

www.yogajournal.com
Yoga Journal teachers directory

www.yogateachersguide.org
Yoga International Magazine teachers guide

acknowledgements

Special thanks to Judith More at Carlton Books for this opportunity, and to Dr Jennifer Golay for her valuable contributions to the book. Thank you to my good-humoured students who posed for all the photos – Holly and Holly, Denise, Cluney, Declan and Marc – and thank you Anna Stevenson for great shots of them! Thanks to Bridget Woods-Kraemer of Yoga Ltd in Cornwall for technical assistance, great classes and real inspiration, and to Sam Armstrong for technical assistance and support on the photo shoot! Thanks to DW Design and Carlton art director Penny Stock for making the book look so good; Tom Marr-Johnson at DJ Freeman for legal support over the years; and to Hilary Whitney for compelling journalism.

Gorgeous colourful clothes courtesy of Nuala and Porselli Dancewear in Covent Garden, London. Mats courtesy of omshop.com.

Special thanks to mates Marc, Wendy, Roz, Holly, Anita, Henry, Norma, Lydia, Trina, Panta and to family – mom, dad, Ron, Randy, Jeff and Barb – for love and laughs. And special, special thanks to Gordon Thomson, Cheryl Liss and Judy Herbert at Body Control Pilates Studio in South Kensington, London, for years of training, and to Shyam and Mira Mehta and to everyone at the Iyengar Yoga Institute, London – and to Geeta Iyengar, Sarah Lytton, Gabriel Halpern, Mark Whitwell, Gurmukh and Baron Baptiste – whose classes I have enjoyed and been inspired by. Thanks to Michael Miller for reminding me about the spiral, and to Sasha Davis for movement extraordinaire! And thanks to John Friend for reminding us to open our hearts and laugh.

about the author

Jill Everett is a certified body-control pilates instructor, certified yoga instructor and founder of Flow Studio in London. Jill's unique style of teaching refelects the influences of classical hatha yoga, precision-alignment Iyengar yoga with props, flowing ashtanga yoga, vini yoga breath and bodywork integration, kundalini yoga energy awareness, anusara yoga's warmth, grace and openess, and pilates' modern updates on balance, core strength, rhythm and alignment. Jill teaches advanced classical pilates matwork and modified pilates preparation exercises for beginners or for those with rehabilitation needs. She also teaches precision-flow yoga classes, yoga therapy and a combination class of pilates and yoga called Pilates Plus. Jill runs yoga and pilates spiritual eco-tourism retreats around the world in beautiful nature reserves in India, Mexico, Maui and Costa Rica where students can experience a simple life living in harmony with nature. If you are interested and would like more information, please contact Jill at www.flowstudio.co.uk or jillneverett@hotmail.com.

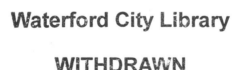